Health and Identity in Egypt

Health and Identity in Egypt

EDITED BY HANIA SHOLKAMY
AND FARHA GHANNAM

The American University in Cairo Press
Cairo   New York

First published in Egypt in 2004 by
The American University in Cairo Press
113 Sharia Kasr el Aini, Cairo, Egypt
420 Fifth Avenue, New York, NY 10018
www.aucpress.com

Dar el Kutub No. 16142/03
ISBN 977 424 833 3

Designed by AUC Press Design Center
Printed in Egypt

Contents

Acknowledgments

The authors would like to acknowledge the support and contributions of Huda Zurayk, Jan Amin, Iman Farid, Noha Gaballah, and Barbara Ibrahim. We also thank the Cairo office of the International Population Council for their moral and administrative support, the government of the Netherlands for its financial support, and the members of the Reproductive Health Working Group for their enthusiasm for this project. This book is dedicated to Dr. Nabil Younis, obstetrician/gynecologist, visionary, researcher, nurturer, and friend.

The Reproductive Health Working Group

The Reproductive Health Working Group (RHWG) is a network of researchers and practitioners from the Arab countries and Turkey united in their commitment to enhance and elaborate current theoretical frameworks and policy directions in the field of reproductive health. The group has been active since 1989 in challenging the narrow focus of population research on fertility control, and has pioneered work in the region on women's reproductive morbidity and on perceptions of health and well-being.

Through a long and close collaboration that has been cemented by comparative and interdisciplinary research, annual meetings, and a series of publications including *The Policy Series on Reproductive Health* (Arabic and English), *Monographs in Reproductive Health* (English), and *Women's Reproduction and Health in Rural Egypt: The Giza Study* by Khattab, H. et al., the RHWG has continued to encourage researchers from the region to view reproductive health through an interdisciplinary lens.

This volume by anthropologists, who are members and/or affiliates of RHWG, addresses the relevance of health perceptions to well-being. While conceived as a regional project, it has been realized as an Egyptian one. Nevertheless this volume reflects the group's keen interest in the importance of social, cultural, and humanistic dimensions of health as a bodily experience.

The RHWG has supported *Health and Identity in Egypt: Shifting Frontiers* through a grant from the government of the Netherlands. The regional office for West Asia and North Africa currently hosts the RHWG and has also contributed its support to this work.

Introduction

FARHA GHANNAM AND HANIA SHOLKAMY

This volume explores the intersection of notions of health and well-being with cultural, class-based, religious, and gender identities in Egypt. The contributors argue that the strategies that men and women adopt to attain health and well-being are also expressions of identity. Anthropologists have addressed the relationship between gender, ideology, political economy, and health, and have commented on how cultural and material resources shape the options and decisions that people make to restore or preserve their health (Early 1982; Morsy 1993; Inhorn 1996). The writers in this collection focus on the significance of health choices, ideals, and experiences to the construction and expression of self and identity. The collation of these chapters was motivated by a desire to describe historical, political, and socioeconomic transformations and processes in Egypt as they have been internalized by individual men and women and expressed in the choices they make in pursuit of well-being. They are written by Arab anthropologists (four Egyptians and a Palestinian) who have worked extensively in Egypt, undertaking their fieldwork predominantly in the late 1990s—the very recent past by ethnographic standards!

This collection views health, well-being, and identity at two levels. First the chapters present experiences of health and fertility or their absence as sites of self and social expression that are charted on the landscape of the body. Thus the papers engage with concepts of class, gender, aesthetics, spirituality, and social stratification through their description of health seeking behavior and of strategies that shape and control/condition the human body.

I

At a second level, these papers engage with identity and well-being as processes of becoming that are actively negotiated, expressed, and reproduced under various socioeconomic and cultural possibilities and constraints. Both identity and well-being are socially experienced fluid notions that change over time and place. Simultaneously, both manifest and structure various practices related to the body. People may feel well in and of themselves but also in accordance with societal and historical constructions of what well-being is. At some moments in time and in some places plumpness implies beauty, health, and strength (Ghannam 1997). In others, being very muscular or very thin is the marker of bodily distinction and of good health.

Perhaps most significantly, the essays in this collection straddle the divide between *being* and *becoming* by addressing identity and well-being as ideals men and women strive to attain. Well-being is not just the status of being in good health but also implies the security of being able to stay that way. People caught in war or in poverty may not actually be suffering from a particular disease or disability but they will feel compromised by their predicament and may not feel able to maintain their well-being. Identity is, similarly, a state of being in the present and a formulation of the future. The papers reflect on the relationship between health and identity as a state of being but one that is profoundly conditioned by peoples' experiences of the past and expectations of the future.

These chapters provide a critique of what we may describe as a western individualistic model of well-being. This model of the individual has pervaded our notions of health and well-being. According to this model, well-being in a biological or biomedical sense means bodily integrity; in a socioeconomic sense it means individual material integrity and sufficiency, and in a political sense it means individual rights and privileges. We recognize this view of the autonomous individual as a compelling one. We also acknowledge that the conditions that engender this view of the individual may well have emanated from European and North American philosophical, political, and socioeconomic traditions but their relations of production have extended beyond the narrow confines of the west and have become a part of other peoples' historical realities. Each paper in this volume can be read as a contribution toward diversifying and challenging the individualized model of well-being. The papers indicate the relevance of socially sanctioned and constructed collective references, which determine the diversity of ideals individuals strive toward. They suggest that health, fertility, and beauty are not absolute and abstract rights, but are socially constructed and collectively defined privileges.

We would like to adopt notions of connectivity and the construction of self as elaborated by Suad Joseph (Joseph 1999, 1993) in her work on the Arab family to situate our own work on identity and well-being. Joseph has joined others in rendering problematic the concept of the autonomous individual as a given of social organization. The individual self is not only enmeshed in a multitude of relationships; it is structured by these relationships. As Joseph puts it, "By connectivity I mean relationships in which a person's boundaries are relatively fluid so that persons feel a part of significant others" (Joseph 1993: 452). Joseph builds on the work of Catherine Keller who envisioned the connected self as a construct, not just as a state of being, but one that implies activity or an intention (Keller 1986: 9; Joseph 1993: 453).

Joseph develops her concept of connectivity in the context of the family and cites patriarchy as the idiom that reproduces connected persons. We would like to consider connectivity in relation to health and well-being. This collection views the activities in which people engage to restore or maintain health, beauty, and fertility as ones which structure connected identities. In this context the self is not the individualist autonomous 'self' assumed by western models. Neither is it the corporatist or collective 'self' associated with Arab societies (Rugh 1984). In this collection a self emerges that is individualized by virtue of its sensual dimension and embodied experiences of health and ill-health. Yet it is also a 'self' in action and in constant mutually constructing conversations with others and with its social and cultural context. It is, as Joseph puts it, "an absorbing and actively defining self and other, each of which shifts as each actor acts" (Joseph 1999: 15). Indeed it is the field of health that brings into focus the duality of the self. For example pain and suffering are individualized experiences but their consequences, cures, and expression are socially and collectively sanctioned and defined.

We posit that health maintenance and pursuits are acts of self-expression and of the construction of intention and identity. They are acts that reflect a connected self that is cognizant of its social, political, and cultural boundaries. They are acts that not only structure a state of being but also create the potentials for a state of becoming.

In this introduction we would like to provide a context in which to place the papers that follow. We shall therefore look briefly at the relevant literature on medical anthropology in the Middle East and on current thinking concerning identity. We shall then revisit individual papers and see how they relate to existing work and how they can be read in the context of relatively new thinking on the social construction of identity and of well-being.

Medical Anthropology as Social Analysis

As far as the medical sciences are concerned, disease and other agents/events that cause ill health (i.e., congenital problems and accidents) are objective realities. Medical therapy restores health, which is defined as the absence of diseases and problems, by addressing the disease or malfunction. Medical anthropology used the logic of medicine by assuming that disease and health are universal objective realities that research "uncovers" and not cultural as well as physical experiences, which are complex and diverse in their meaning and interpretation (Foucault 1976; Wartovsky 1976; Comaroff 1978; Foster and Anderson 1978; Eisenberg and Kleinman 1981; Worsley 1982: 315, 327; Young 1982; Good 1994). Anthropologists described cultural variations in the management of diseases and employed biomedical categories in defining a condition of ill-health, while anthropological theories were employed in the description of how indigenous peoples behaved when afflicted with such a condition.

The Explanatory Model of Illness approach appeared on the anthropological scene to focus on the social and experiential particularities of illness and healing (Good 1977; Kleinman 1980; Eisenberg and Kleinman 1981). This approach located a degree of confusion in anthropology in connection with the concepts used to describe health and ill-health. Its proponents therefore attempted to redefine and refine key terms in the area of medical anthropology. While 'disease' was defined as the arena of the biomedical mode, 'illness' became the person's experience of the ignoble condition of being not healthy. 'Sickness' was the category that covers both terms (Young 1982: 264). With these new concepts the Explanatory Model of Illness school differentiated between the biomedical approach, which focuses on disease, and the anthropological view, which recognizes the distinction between the disease and the person's experience of it.

The Explanatory Model approach emphasized the relevance of peoples' culturally constructed experience of disease. However, it failed to account for the conditions that produce ill health. The school's focus on illness and adaptation led to its neglect of the consequences of peoples' social, political, and economic conditions to health and ill-health (Young 1982: 276).

The politico-economic perspective on health, also referred to as Critical Medical Anthropology, emerged to stress the interaction between macro-level conditions and the health experiences and problems of individuals and communities. Critical Medical Anthropology defined 'illness' as the individualized experience of ill health, and 'sickness' as the process through which experienced symptoms are given socially recognizable meaning. 'Disease' retained its biomedical meaning. This school of thought focuses on the social relations that produce the forms and distribution of ill health, or, as they would call it, of sickness. Besides the obvious link between poverty and ill-health, critical medical anthropology called attention to the relationship between health and power in society and examined sickness as an expression of powerlessness. The lens of political economy has located asymmetry in the interaction between patient and doctor, and posited social class and power relations as important factors in the seemingly neutral process of disease diagnosis (Onoge 1975; Morsy 1978, 1990).

As far as therapy is concerned, Critical Medical Anthropology recognizes that the science of physical things, including biomedicine, is part of the political ideology of the dominant west. As such, modern medicine was seen as more than just an effective science. Biomedicine was seen to contribute to the mystification of the human power-relationships that are articulated in states of sickness and in therapy (Onoge 1975; Morsy 1978, 1990, 1993; Frankenberg 1980; Taussig 1980; Navarro 1981, 1986; Young 1982; Singer 1989). Physicians not only cure, but they also impose a way of thinking and behaving and thereby enforce hierarchical relations in society. Their dislike of alternative and indigenous medical traditions was interpreted as a contest between different ideologies, in contrast to the way many physicians see it, namely as a preference for knowledge over ignorance (Worsley 1982; Morsy 1990).

The above brief consideration of the evolution of medical anthropology shows how the interpretation of health and ill-health progressed from a strict focus on the disease to an interest in its cultural context and then to a consideration of the macro-level conditions that produce health and ill-health.

The notion of well-being is a relatively new one. Enshrined by the World Health Organization (WHO) as a human right, well-being remains an elusive concept. According to the WHO, "Health is a state of complete physical, mental, and social well-being and not merely the absence of disease or infirmity" (WHO 2000). This definition sets high standards that few people in the world can attain. This definition of health affirms that being healthy is far more than just being not sick. Biology is not the only factor or variable that shapes health; social, economic, and political as well as cultural ones are also relevant. Indeed it is these factors, which structure the domain that is beyond biology, that very domain that we have come to know as well-being.

The distance between the residual category called health (the absence of disease and disability) and the ideal of well-being is a problematic one. Few in this world can realize the mandate of WHO. But in every society, community, and family there are conditions and structures that are deemed essential for and conducive to well-being; ones that reach beyond medically measurable health and structure well-being. The following essays are about this domain as it is defined and experienced in Egypt at the present. The essays are not about disease conditions per se. They are about fertility, beauty, serenity, peace of mind, energy, and ability. All are indicators of well-being, all are located in the perceived future but contingent on the present, all are embodied ideals that are shaped by social, cultural, material, and political forces and all are experiences that relate to health but express identity and social self-hood.

Farha Ghannam looks at the topic of weight and well-being and introduces social, cultural, and aesthetic factors, which diversify the western model of ideal weight and ideal beauty. She also illustrates the relationship between health, identity, and well-being in specific cultural and socioeconomic contexts. Other papers in this collection de-link health from well-being and illustrate how health as the domain of biology can become contingent on socially defined well-being. Not only is the distinction between the two in terms of sociology and biology, the distance is also temporal. If health is a state of being, then well-being can be viewed as a state conditioned by the potentiality of becoming or remaining healthy. In this collection we are looking at states of being and of becoming healthy.

The papers in this collection engage gendered power and hierarchy in their analysis of health and well-being. They do so by privileging individual agency and subjective experiences of a connected and contextualized self. Phenomenology provides the tools necessary for understanding the self's experiences of health. Phenomenologists argue that life experiences and trajectory imply that there is a subjective dimension to ill-health and health, which lies beyond the scope of impersonal science.

This premise is distinct from the issue of the cultural construction of disease widely discussed by the Explanatory Model of Illness. There is a difference between the study of peoples' reactions to predefined conditions and the proposition of the possibility of subjective and cultural variation in the conditions themselves. Phenomenologists stress individual and cultural construction as an aspect of the subjective creation of meaning (Young 1982; Myntti 1983; Lock and Gordon 1988). They argue that there is such a thing as 'embodied knowing' as well as 'abstract knowing.' In view of this hypothesis, health perceptions are therefore how we translate physical experiences into social and emotional ones. This process references gender, power, and social positions, which are all historical constructs (Duroche 1990).

Ghannam focuses on the female body as the site for the expression of cultural and class identities. She also stresses the interrelationship between body, mind, and society (Scheper-Hughes and Lock 1987: 6; Turner 1992; Saltonstall 1993). Ghannam shows how culture and society shape the female body and how women, through their bodies, engage with their social world. The important concept that she present as far as health is concerned is that of the body as the arena where knowledge is experienced and reconstituted.

All the papers in this volume reflect this theoretical genealogy in one way or another. We read in this collection about the interrelationship between class and etiologies of diseases and health seeking behavior (Kamal); on the relationship between culture, aesthetics, and the body (Ghannam); and on the confluence of culture, community, history, and fertility (Sholkamy). But these papers also engage with another body of literature, one concerning the social construction of individual and collective identity. In the following section we shall attempt to see the relevance of our work to recent writings on identity.

Identity: Shifting Meanings

Struggles over notions of well-being cannot be separate from individual and collective identities, which are important bases from which people create new activities, new worlds, and new ways of being (Holland et al. 1998: 5). The drastic shift in studies of identity was marked by a rejection of the determinism of biology in the construction of enduring identities such as those of gender and race. Identity came to be viewed as a product of historical, socioeconomic, political, and cultural forces and not as an inevitable result of physical determinants. This later approach, which has been loosely labeled as social constructionism, emphasized that identity is constructed through the eyes of the other and is the product of interaction between individuals and institutions (Calhoun 1994; Jenkins 1996). This theoretical move is best exemplified in the study of the self and how it changed over time. During the 1970s, two main approaches (naturalist and culturist) in anthropological literature aimed to analyze the self. The naturalist approach focused on a universal self, which is primarily a complex of natural, species-given structures and processes (Holland et al. 1998: 20). The other approach (culturalist in its orientation) argued that the self is shaped mainly by culture, and its advocates worked to explore selves in different societies. In the late 1970s and early 1980s, social constructionists, who focused especially on criticizing the assumption that there was an essential self, a durable organization of the mind/body, questioned both these approaches (27). They particularly criticized the culturalist tendency to view the self as a fixed and changeless entity that is formed during childhood and that mirrored the values of a particular culture.

Social constructionists are most informative in their rejection of the conceptualization of identity as a given natural entity and as a product of individual will (Calhoun 1994). Social constructionism, however, is strongly criticized for granting determining power to social structures while granting little agency to social actors. The emphasis on socialization and the power of society in structuring individual and collective identities leads many social constructionists to treat identities in terms nearly as essentialist as those of biological determinists (Calhoun 1994: 16). Social constructionists are accused of depicting identity as a coherent, unified, fixed product that is shaped by various socioeconomic factors such as class, gender, and race. They also tend to suggest that there is a solid essence that determines collective and individual identity, which leads them to emphasize stability and eliminate contradictions.

New social movements, women's movements, gay groups, civil rights movements, and anti-colonial movements in the Third World promoted a critical discussion of the concept of identity and its theorization (Rutherford 1990; Stuarty 1993; Calhoun 1994; Somers and Gibson 1994; Sarup 1996). Through struggles for political recognition and personal validation, these movements questioned the dominant view of identity as a coherent, unitary, and stable entity.

These struggles shifted the attention to the analysis of identity "as contradictory, as composed of more than one discourse, as composed always across the silences of the other, as written in and through ambivalence and desire" (Hall 1991: 49). Several authors shifted the attention from a stable and changeless identity into conceptualizing identifications as "never completed, never finished; that they are always as subjectivity itself is, in process" (Hall 1991: 47). As Richard Jenkins (1996: 4) emphasizes, "[i]dentity can in fact only be understood as process. As being or becoming. One's social identity . . . is never a final or settled matter" (see also Calhoun 1994; Moore 1994). In short, identities are dynamic and contextual processes that are shaped by a multiplicity of forces and discourses (Rutherford 1990; Calhoun 1994; Moore 1994).

Feminism and Gender Analysis

Feminist anthropology has provided ample documentation of the permeation of power inequalities between men and women. In general, feminist anthropologists pursued the gender bias in communities and institutions, and described the disadvantaged position of women especially in economic and political spheres. Feminist scholars pointed out the bias implicit in the identification of women with nature and reproduction, while men were extolled as the creators of culture. This divide had served to legitimate the inferior position of women in societies. Feminist anthropologists scrutinized what they saw as a fallacy, and questioned the divide between nature and culture and the corresponding mapping of genders to this divide (Mathieu 1978; MacCormack and Strathern 1980; cf. Ortner 1974). They illustrated how this symbolic opposition between nature and culture had reflected on social relations and had contributed to the reproduction of gender hierarchies. Meanwhile, others were questioning the universality of this dualism in the first place (Collier and Rosaldo 1981; Harris 1981; Moore 1988: 25).

The feminist interest in women's health came subsequent to this focus on power relations between genders. The problematic relationship between modern medicine and women was taken up by Emily Martin in her book, *The Woman in the Body: A Cultural Analysis of Reproduction* (1989). Here she presents the views of American women whom she interviewed on their experiences of their own reproductive health and sickness. Martin questions the validity of medical hypothesis that pretend to be unbiased. She maintains that medical metaphors, as expressed in medical textbooks, are culturally specific and consequently are very much party to the gender biases and the power relations of the social and intellectual contexts from which they evolve (Martin 1989: 40).

Martin subjects 'biomedical perceptions' of women's health to a feminist scrutiny. She shows how biomedical interpretations are only one possibility of explaining medical facts (52). She also illustrates that scientific metaphors of reproduction serve the purposes of the medical institution rather than favoring the interest of women (66). She explains that medicine is a product of the economic and political order of the west. As proof she mentions that medical metaphors derive from images of commodity capitalism. Consequently biomedicine describes menstruation as 'failed production' and menopause is characterized as a kind of 'failure of the authority structure of the body.' Both metaphors imply that menopause and menstruation are negative experiences (45). Left to their own interpretations, women themselves may not necessarily define menstruation and menopause as negative events in their lives.

Martin shows how gender relations and their power disequilibria permeate medical discourse. Others have continued her line of investigation (Jacobus, Keller, and Shuttleworth 1990).[1] On the whole, the work of gender-sensitive analysts is still making its mark in the field of health and ill-health. It is also paving the way for research that sees health not only as an interaction between disease or disability and the individual, but as a social and political situation where the gendered understanding and experiences of individuals and communities define and shape people's concepts of health.

Collective identities such as those based on class, race, and nationalism are no longer viewed as ready-made homogenous totalities. Many studies have illustrated the inner contradictions and divisions of these identities. Recent studies, for instance, have challenged the previous emphasis of the political left on class as a structuring force that determines the views and practices of individuals. Identity, these studies show, cannot be reduced to the single logic of class (Rutherford 1990: 19). Class often intersects with race, gender, nationalism, and religion in the formation of individual and collective identities.

Looking at how gendered identities have been conceptualized over the past three decades can best capture the previous shifts. For a long time women's inferior status was assumed to be the result of physical or

---

1. For further gender-informed analysis on women and health see Petchesky 1984, Stern 1986, and Roberts 1991.

biological characteristics (especially reproductive functions). Since the 1960s, however, feminists have to a large extent succeeded in separating sex from gender, and argued that the source of women's subordination is not biology but the social construction of sexual differences (Moore 1994). Rather than grounding inequality in natural biological differences that are assumed to be universal, fixed, and unchangeable, gender allowed feminists to analyze distinctions between men and women as the product of social and political relationships (Waylen 1996: 6). Viewing gender as a social construct that varies through time and space meant that gender inequalities could be challenged and transformed (6). In their struggle, however, feminists suppressed differences between women and reproduced some of the universalist claims that they tried to question (Stuarty 1990: 34). Women from different classes, races, and ages were all grouped under the same label: woman. An essence was assumed to determine an identity that women shared despite their cultures and social classes. In the 1980s, Third World women, women of color, and some feminists questioned the label 'woman' and criticized it as a unitary and ahistorical category (Waylen 1996: 7). Studies proliferated to show that there are significant differences between women's experiences in various contexts. The emphasis, however, was on cross-cultural variations, and gendered identities continued to be seen as a direct consequence of exposure to and compliance with cultural categories and the straightforward outcome of biological categories (Moore 1994: 54).

During the late 1980s, post-structuralists succeeded in drawing attention to the ways in which masculinity and femininity are constructed in the individual subject rather than seeing gender as a set of roles into which people are socialized (Waylen 1996: 6). Psychoanalysis has also been influential in questioning notions of identity and in showing that each is formed of multiple and competing discourses, which challenge any efforts to attain stable self-recognition or coherent subjectivity (Calhoun 1994: 20). The analysis shifted to how the subject is constructed, and identity became viewed increasingly as the interplay between class, race, gender, sexuality, and other elements. Identity is a crucial aspect of subjectivity and subjectivity is perhaps best understood as a project, as something always under construction, never perfect (20). A subject, recent writings show, has a plurality of identities, and individual actors are often entangled in multiple and contradictory individual and social identities (Rutherford 1990; Stuarty 1990; Giddens 1991; Jenkins 1996; Calhoun 1994). The attention is increasingly directed to the theorization of how individuals become gendered subjects; that is, how they come to have representations of themselves as women and men, to make representations of others, and to organize their social practices in such a way as to reproduce dominant categories, discourses, and practices (Moore 1994: 51).

Rather than a simple opposition between essentialism and constructionism, the papers in this volume map various strategies and possibilities for analyzing issues related to identity and well-being. The papers address several important questions: Is identity always so fragmented and fluid as suggested in recent studies? Are various identities, especially gender, fluid and flexible to the same extent? How is identity related to embodiment? How do social agents (a low-income female college student in Cairo, a possessed woman in a working-class neighborhood, or a childless woman in Upper Egypt) negotiate various social norms and regulations in the making of their bodies and identities? How do these agents articulate contradictory discourses, desires, and feelings in the construction of a beautiful figure, socially valued identity, and a healthy body? How are notions of well-being grasped, manifested, internalized, and transformed by social actors?

This volume tries to challenge various stereotypes about the region. Most papers shift attention from the usual emphasis on Islam as the determining factor in shaping gender identities to examine the complex local, national, and global forces that shape bodies and identities. Drawing on narratives, observations, personal experience, questionnaires, and structured interviews, these papers reveal part of the interplay between individual and collective identities such as national, religious, class-based, and gender identities and how this interplay shapes notions of well-being. The various papers examine well-being and identity as processes of becoming that are never finalized or finished. They explore struggles over identity and well-being by looking at issues such as justice, illness practices, beauty, and somatization. The authors contribute to current studies of identity and well-being by addressing two interrelated issues: firstly, globalization, embodiment, and self-identity, and, secondly, sexuality, justice, and dignity.

Globalization, Embodiment, and Self-identity

Embodiment, as the various papers show, is central to both identity and well-being. The body, how it is represented and maintained, communicates various issues related to self-identity. As argued by several authors, "[s]ocial identification in isolation from embodiment is unimaginable

(Jenkins 1996: 21). The papers in this volume vary in the emphasis they place on the forces that structure identity and shape embodiment. Drawing on Pierre Bourdieus' concepts of habitus and fields, Montasser M. Kamal makes a strong case for how class structures illness practices and self-identity in Cairo.

Narratives of middle-class informants show the strong link between views of self-identification, embodiment, and the socioeconomic status. Kamal argues persuasively that class consciousness and identity enabled his informant to recreate boundaries between the self as educated petty bourgeoisie and the perceived "other as a homogenous (relatively) lower class." Ayman, a young man with a middle-class background, does not want to go to a doctor who caters to the poor. He prefers to go to a private clinic attended only by people 'like him.' In his encounter with the doctor, Ayman makes sure that he presents his body (by wearing fancy clothing, shaving, and using nice cologne) in ways that confirm his class background and that signal his respectable family background. Similarly, to express her distinction, Amina, a middle-class woman, inserts English words when she describes complications with her pregnancy. Words such as 'bleeding,' 'anaemia,' and 'fibroma' became part of her encounters with doctors and discussions with friends.

Although Kamal chooses to emphasize class as a structuring force, the rich narratives in his paper provide clear indications as to how gender and age also play central roles in shaping the habitus of social agents and in shaping their views of health. Masculinity, for example, comes out as a strong factor that shapes self-identity and views of well-being. Thus, Ayman, who was doing his military service, describes his hesitation about telling other men in the camp about his illness. "If I tell anyone," Ayman says, "it will spread and they will all make fun of me and talk behind me and in front of me about 'being like a girl.'" In addition to his middle-class status, Ayman is clearly asserting his masculine identity by avoiding any signs of femininity. Power relationships in the family also shape how social actors react and view their health and well-being. This was clear with Amina who does not tell her husband and mother about complications with her pregnancy because she feels that her body is the cause of tension between her husband and mother. Her husband, she feared, was going to think that she did not want to have his baby while her mother was going to blame her son-in-law for using Amina's body as a "container" to bear children.

In addition to class, other papers pay close attention to gender, age, and education in the formation of identity and notions of well-being.

They show how globalization is shaping identities, views of the body, and well-being, as shown too in the various studies in this volume. Ghannam's paper illuminates aspects of what Anthony Giddens calls the self as "reflexive project" (1991: 32). In late modernity and with the growing globalization of culture, Giddens argues that self identity has to be routinely created and sustained in the reflexive activities of the individual (52). The flows of information, images, discourses, and goods are providing new possibilities for individuals to shape their bodies and identities in different ways. For example, as shown in Ghannam's paper, the presence of new creams and dyes are enabling young women in low-income districts of Cairo to acquire lighter skin color and blond hair.

Various scholars have been trying to understand the social, political, and cultural factors that shape women's views of their bodies and identities (Bordo 1995). Eating disorders, in particular, such as anorexia, bulimia, and compulsive eating are attracting the attention of many researchers, especially in the west (Caskey 1986; Epstein 1987; Banks 1992; Hesse-Biber 1996; Garrett 1998). Such studies are still largely lacking in the Middle East. Ghannam conveys part of the pressures and struggles that women are negotiating in the formation of their bodies in Cairo. There is a growing obsession (especially among middle and upper-middle classes) with the thin body. This obsession is manifested in the proliferation of discourses in the media, the increasing number of weight-loss clinics, and the growing appetite suppressants sold in supermarkets and pharmacies.

Sexuality, Justice, and Dignity

The papers also address the interplay between sexual desire, agency, and notions of justice. This is most clearly reflected in the papers written by Heba El-Kholy and Hania Sholkmay. El-Kholy examines spirit possession as a pervasive and potent discourse among women in low-income Cairo for the expression of unconventional views on often taboo subjects. She argues that spirit possession is a commentary on two important broader socioeconomic and political changes that shape women's lives. First, it is a critique of the attempts of the media and community leaders to Islamize women's behaviors (through veiling, praying, reading the Qur'an, and so on). Spirits hinder the attempts of women to follow Islamic norms and push them to non-Islamic actions such as drinking beer. Second, spirit possession is a commentary on the inability of the man to satisfy his wife sexually and to provide for her financially. Possessed women, El-Kholy tells us, expressed a consistent lack of sexual desire. Spirit possession becomes central to resolving the conflict that results between Islamic regulation, which instructs women to obey their husband's sexual demands, and the women's lack of sexual desire. Spirits force women to reject marriage proposals, improper sexual requests, and sexual intercourse with their husbands. In this context, spirit possession becomes 'a discourse of resistance.'

Utilizing Victor Turner's (1967, 1988) concepts of communitas and liminality, Hania Sholkamy shows how cultural concepts such as an infertility spell (*mushahra*) are linked to individual and collective identities. *Mushahra* is based on the belief that any woman can be the victim of a spell that may prevent pregnancy. This belief, according to Sholkamy, creates a constant channel of mobility from statuses of fertile to infertile, and vice versa. The social significance of the spell is that it places all women under the same rules, the same codes of practices. The belief that all women and their female relatives are subject to the same threat becomes a powerful way to counter the social stigmas and consequences (such as divorce or polygamy) of infertility. This notion, Sholkamy suggests, establishes a sense of equality between women and is linked to a more general notion of justice.

Conclusion

A reader of the following chapters will find a number of common themes and what we hope are contributions to our understanding of the region and its peoples. Papers in this collection challenge lingering stereotypes of Egyptian men and women. By stereotypes we mean the taken-for-granted assumptions about daily life and people in Egypt. These are assumptions that have not been revisited recently and reassessed in view of how people master their lives and destinies. Rather than focus on impoverished nutrition, we look at the bodily images and ideals of middle-class and less-well-to-do women and men. In another chapter we learn of poor rural women's concerns for values—which we tend to associate with modern developed democracies rather than poor and marginal rural communities—such as those of justice and of equality (Sholkamy).

We learn of urban women's very secular and pragmatic engagement with the world of spirits, and how even these otherworldly beings are subjected to the power and social relationships within which women are enmeshed (El-Kholy). We learn about the struggle of middle-class men and women to achieve ideals of health and well-being while maintaining their distinction and separation from other (lower) classes (Kamal). Thus the essays focus on lived reality, and favor ethnography while extending critical reflection to the descriptions and ethnographic accounts. As a result they illustrate the integration of events and experiences that tend to be reified by analysis. All the chapters provide accessible stories of how fluid these concepts, attributes, experiences, and conditions are, and how any adequate understanding of people and communities demands an appreciation of this fluidity.

The chapters claim space for agency and individual initiative. They show how men and women are active in shaping their bodies and constructing their individual and connected identities for themselves and for others. The pursuit of health and bodily ideals is a path paved with diverse and sometimes conflicting choices. We make choices on our own behalf and on behalf of others in deciding, for example, between different medical traditions, resources, and doctors. While health and ill-health are shaped by forces and by societal and biological determinants, it would be a mistake to forgo (connected) individual and collective choices and initiative. The essays in these chapters clearly address both determinants and agency and so relay the rich and complex character of identity and well-being as lived experiences.

Bibliography

Banks, Caroline Giles, 1992, "Culture in Culture-Bound Syndromes: The Case of Anorexia Nervosa," *Social Science and Medicine*, 34 (8), 867–84.

Bordo, Susan, 1995, *Unbearable Weight: Feminism, Western Culture, and the Body*. Berkeley: University of California Press.

Calhoun, Craig, ed., 1994, *Social Theory and the Politics of Identity*. Oxford: Basil Blackwell.

Caskey, Noelle, 1986, "Interpreting Anorexia Nervosa," *The Female Body in Western Culture*, Susan Rubin Suleiman, ed., 175–192. Cambridge: Harvard University Press.

Cohen, Anthony P., 1994, *Self Consciousness: An Alternative Anthropology of Identity*. London: Routledge.

Duroche, Leonard L., 1990, "Male Perception as Social Construct," *Men, Masculinity, and Social Theory*, Jeff Hearn and David Morgan, eds, 170–185. London: Unwin & Hyman.

Early, Evelyn A., 1982, "The Logic of Well Being: Therapeutic Narratives in Cairo, Egypt," *Social Science and Medicine*, 16 (16): 1491–1497.

Eisenberg, Leon, and Arthur Kleinman, 1981, "Clinical Social Science: Is Medicine Impeded by Too Much Science?" *The Relevance of Social Science for Medicine*, Leon Eisenberg and Arthur Klienman, eds., 1–23. Dordrecht: D. Reidel Publishing Company.

Epstein, B., 1987, "Women's Anger and Compulsive Eating," *Fed Up and Hungry*, M. Lawrence, ed. London: The Women's Press.

Foucault, Michel, 1975, *The Birth of the Clinic: An Archeology of Medical Perception*. New York: Vintage Books.

Frankenberg, R., 1980, "Medical Anthropology and Development: A Theoretical Perspective," *Social Science and Medicine*, 14B: 197–207.

Garrett, Catherine, 1998, *Beyond Anorexia: Narrative, Spirituality and Recovery*. Cambridge: Cambridge University Press.

Ghannam, Farha, 1997, "Fertile, Plump, and Strong: The Social Construction of the Female Body in Low Income Cairo." Monograph. Cairo: The Reproductive Health Working Group, Population Council.

Giddens, Anthony, 1991, "Modernity and Self-Identity: Self and Society," *Late Modern Age*. Stanford: Stanford University Press.

Good, Byron, 1994, *Medicine, Rationality, and Experience: An Anthropological Perspective*. Cambridge: Cambridge University Press.

———, 1977, "The Heart of What's the Matter," *Culture, Medicine, and Psychiatry*, 1: 25–58.

Hall, Stuart, 1991a, "The Local and the Global: Globalization and Ethnicity," *Culture, Globalization and the World-System*, Anthony D. King, ed., 19–39. Binghamton: State University of New York Press.

———, 1991b, "Old and New Identities, Old and New Ethnicities," *Culture, Globalization, and the World-System*, Anthony D. King, ed., 41–68. Binghamton: State University of New York Press.

Hesse-Biber, Sharlene Janice, 1996, *Am I Thin Enough Yet? The Cult of Thinness and the Commercialization of Identity*. Oxford: Oxford University Press.

Holland, Dorothy, William Lachicotte Jr., Debra Skinner, and Carole Cain, 1998, *Identity and Agency in Cultural Worlds*. Cambridge: Harvard University Press.

Inhorn, Marcia Claire, 1996, *Infertility and Patriarchy: The Cultural Politics of Gender and Family Life in Egypt*. Philadelphia: University of Pennsylvania Press.

———, 1994, *Quest for Conception: Gender, Infertility, and Egyptian Medical Traditions*. Philadelphia: University of Pennsylvania Press.

Jacobu, Mary, Evelyn Fox Keller, and Sally Shuttleworth, 1990, *Body/Politics: Women and the Discourse of Science*. New York: Routledge.

Jenkins, Richard, 1996, *Social Identity*. London: Routledge.

Joseph, Suad, 1999, *Intimate Selving in Arab Families: Gender, Self, and Identity*. Syracuse: Syracuse University Press.

————, 1993, "Gender and Relationality among Arab Families in Lebanon," *Feminist Studies*, 19 (3): 465–486.

Kelleher, David and Sheila Hillier, eds., 1996, *Researching Cultural Differences in Health*. New York: Routledge.

Keller, Catherine, 1986, *From a Broken Web: Separation, Sexism, and Self*. Boston: Beacon Press.

Kleinman, Arthur, 1980, *Patients and Healers in the Context of Culture: An Exploration of the Borderland between Anthropology, Medicine, and Psychiatry*. Berkeley: University of California Press.

Lewis, I.M. and A. Al-Safi, and S. Hurreiz, 1991, *Women's Medicine: The Zar Bori Cult in Africa and Beyond*. Edinburgh: Edinburgh University Press for the International African Institute.

Lock, Margaret and Deborah Gordon, eds., 1988, *Biomedicine Examined*. Boston: Kluwer Acedemic Publishers.

MacCormack, Carol P. Marelyn Strathern, 1980, *Nature, Culture, and Gender*. Cambridge: Cambridge University Press.

Mach, Zdzislaw, 1993, *Symbols, Conflict, and Identity: Essays in Political Anthropology*. Albany: State University of New York Press.

Moore, Henrietta L., 1994, *A Passion for Difference*. Bloomington: Indiana University Press.

Morsy, Soheir A., 1993, *Gender, Sickness, and Healing in Rural Egypt: Ethnography in Historical Context*. Boulder: Westview Press.

————, 1990, "Political Economy in Medical Anthropology," Medical Anthropology: *A Handbook of Theory and Method*, Thomas M. Johnson and Carolyn F. Sargent, eds., 26–46. New York: Greenwood Press.

————, 1978, "Sex Roles, Power, and Illness in an Egyptian Village," *American Anthropologist*, 5 (1): 137–150.

————, 1978, "Sex Differences and Folk Illness in an Egyptian," *Women in the Muslim World*, op. cit.

Myntti, Cynthia, 1985, "Changing Attitudes towards Health: Some Observations from the Hujariya," *Economy, Society, and Culture in Contemporary Yemen*, B.R. Pridham, ed., 165–171. London: Croom Helm.

Navarro, V., 1981, *Imperialism, Health and Medicine*. Farmingdale: Baywood.

Onoge, Omafume, 1975, "Capitalism and Public Health: A Neglected Theme in the Medical Anthropology of Africa," *Topias and Utopias in Health*, Stanley R. Ingman and Anthony E. Thomas, eds. The Hague: Mouton.

Ortner, Sherry B., 2001, "Is Female to Male as Nature is to Culture," *Feminism and the Study of Religion: A Reader*, Darlene M. Juschka, ed., 61–80. New York: Continuum.

———, 1974, "Is Female to Male as Nature to Culture?" *Women, Culture, and Society*, M. Rosaldo and L. Lamphere, eds., 67–87. Stanford: Stanford University Press.

Paige, Jeffery M., 1975, *Agrarian Revolution: Social Movements and Export Agriculture in the Underdeveloped World*. New York: Free Press.

Rugh, Andrea B., 1984, *Family in Contemporary Egypt*. Syracuse: Syracuse University Press.

Rutherford, Jonathan, 1990, "A Place Called Home: Identity and the Cultural Politics of Difference," *Identity: Community, Culture, Difference*, Jonathan Rutherford, ed., 9–27. London: Lawrence and Wishart.

Saltonstall, Robin, 1993, "Healthy Bodies, Social Bodies: Men's and Women's Concepts and Practices of Health in Everyday Life," *Social Science* 36 (1): 7–15.

Sarup, Madan, 1996, *Identity, Culture, and the Postmodern World*. Athens: The University of Georgia Press.

Scheper-Hughes, Nancy and Margaret M. Lock, 1987, "The Mindful Body: A Prolegomenon to Future Work in Medical Anthropology," *Medical Anthropology Quarterly*, 1 (1): 16–41.

Singer, M., 1989, "The Coming of Age of Critical Medical Anthropology," Social Science and Medicine, 28 (11): 1193–1203.

Somers, Margaret R. and Gloria D. Gibson, 1994, *Reclaiming the Epistemological "Other": Narrative and the Social Construction of Identity in Social Theory and the Politics of Identity*, Craig Calhoun, ed., 37–99. Oxford: Basil Blackwell.

Stuarty, Andrea, 1990, "Feminism: Dead or Alive," *Identity: Community, Culture, Difference*, Jonathan Rutherford, ed., 28–42. London: Lawrence & Wishart.

Taussig, M., 1980, "Reification and the Consciousness of the Patient," *Social Science and Medicine*, 14B: 3–13.

Turner, Bryan S., 1992, *Regulating Bodies: Essays in Medical Sociology*. New York: Routledge.

Waylen, Georgina, 1996, *Gender in Third World Politics*. Boulder: Lynne Rienner.

Wolf, Eric R., 1969, *Peasant Wars of the Twentieth Century*. New York: Harper & Row.

Worsley, Peter, 1982, "Non-Western Medical Systems," *Annual Review of Anthropology*, 11: 315–348.

Young, Allen, 1982, "The Anthropology of Illness and Sickness," *Annual Review of Anthropology*, 11: 257–285.

A Discourse of Resistance

Spirit Possession among Women in Low-income Cairo

HEBA EL-KHOLY

This chapter is about spirit possession as a form of expression among low-income women in Cairo.[1] It is also about how they construct awareness of their selves, of gender relations, and of their position in society. This forms part of a larger study dealing with women's 'every day' forms of resistance. The aim of the larger study is to capture the texture of women's daily conflicts and negotiation strategies, both in the household and in the labor market. The focus of this particular paper is on two areas contested by women—sexual relations and encroaching 'Islamization'—and on the form of expression through which these issues are most vividly articulated and challenged—spirit possession.

The chapter is divided into four sections. In the first section, I frame my arguments and data within a broader theoretical discussion of resistance, consciousness, and gender relations. I then go on to elaborate the argument that spirit possession represents a discourse of resistance, a language of protest. The beliefs expressed through the idiom of possession, its episodes, images, and ritualized ceremonies, the *zar* and *hadra*, are best understood as 'infrapolitics,' a "type of resistance that dare not speak in its own name" (Scott 1985: 20). In the third section, I illustrate this argument by focusing on two of the recurrent 'themes' that came out of my in-depth interviews: religion and sex. In the fourth section, I explore the limitations of spirit possession as a discourse of resistance for women.

---

1. This paper was first presented at the panel discussion on Gender and the Indigenization of Knowledge, Sixth Congress of the International Association of Middle Eastern Studies, Mafrak, Jordan, April 10–14, 1996.

Resistance, Consciousness, and Gender Relations

Traditional Marxist approaches to resistance and consciousness are inadequate for a culturally and historically sensitive understanding of the dynamics of gender relations. Instead, I argue for adopting the concept of "everyday resistance" to better capture women's diverse forms of active, subtle and passive protest and negotiation. The term 'everyday' in relation to forms of resistance, coined by James Scott in 1985 with particular reference to the peasantry, is used to capture a wide range of contestary actions and behaviors of subordinate groups, in between open, collective revolt and passive consent. These include actions such as foot dragging, tax evasion, avoidance protest, sabotage, gossip, slander, feigned ignorance, etc. (Scott 1985, 1986).

Studies of resistance have traditionally been dominated by accounts of open confrontations in the form of large-scale rebellions and revolutions, and have largely focused on class conflict as the major cause of struggle (Wolf 1969). Influenced largely by a narrow Marxist paradigm, resistance has been viewed mainly as an organized struggle by subordinate groups informed by a coherent oppositional ideology, and focusing specifically on the working class. A critical assumption in Marxist theory regarding resistance is the relationship between positionality and consciousness, a relationship which emphasizes the split between 'objective' conditions of oppression and 'subjective' consciousness of this oppression, between ideology and behavior, between the economic and the political spheres (McLellan 1973). This model of struggle, and its relationship to power and consciousness is also implicit in the model adopted by early feminists in the west, with its emphasis on 'consciousness raising' as an essential strategy.

The last ten years, however, have given way to a broader usage of the concept of resistance, largely as a backlash against the narrow, economistic, and gender-blind interpretations of Marxist theories of power. The opening up of new possibilities for understanding power and resistance has been influenced by feminist theory and practice as well as by the post-structuralist/post-modernist critique, with Michel Foucault's work assuming particular importance. With post-structuralism the margins between the objective and the subjective began to fade and the concept of false consciousness lost much of its earlier force. Consciousness is no longer being sought in overt and explicit statements "of common predicament on the part of a social group, but also in the implicit language of symbolic activity" (Comaroff 1987: 192). Dominant social structures are no longer being viewed as independent and monolithic entities that are challenged only during dramatic instances of revolt, but rather as a web of contradictory processes that are continuously being renegotiated and contested (Haynes and Prakash 1991). As Scott convincingly argued in *Weapons of the Weak*, a history focused only on the exceptional occasions of mass revolts and rebellions would tell us little about the more durable day-to-day struggles of subordinate groups. These daily protests and struggles "do not throw up the manifestos, demonstrations, and pitched battles that normally compel attention, but vital territory is being won and lost here too" (Scott 1986: 6).

Despite criticisms by various scholars (Turton 1986; Prakash and Haynes 1991; White 1986), the concept of "everyday forms of resistance" nonetheless remains a valuable analytic tool and is supported by recent theorizing about the nature of power.[2] The works of Foucault and Antonio Gramsci have been particularly influential in this debate. These works have highlighted the significance of ideological practices in power and resistance, and have called for an appreciation of the connections between physical coercion and violence, and ideological instruments of domination; between legality and force and more subtle consensual norms (Abu-Lughod 1990). Moreover, the importance of moving beyond a strictly economic analysis of resistance that focuses on 'material' struggles such as wages, rent, land, etc., to less explored areas like popular culture, for example, is now acknowledged (Turton 1986; Haynes and Prakash 1991).

Applying the concept of 'everyday' resistance to the study of gender relations would illuminate the diverse ways in which gender-based hierarchies are continuously being contested and negotiated, reveal the diverse and often subtle expressions of women's 'consciousness,' as well as expose the specific instruments, tactics, and modalities of power underlying gender relations. This approach has the potential of revealing women as they live their daily lives with all its contradictions: as neither passive victims of oppression, nor as all-powerful actors, as they are often portrayed in studies of gender relations in the Middle East.

Moreover, an understanding of the potentially consequential acts of everyday resistance is an essential complement to the emerging

---

2. For a discussion of the various attempts to define power, the difficulties of agreeing on one definition, and how such definitions reflect different people's interest in both the outcomes and the locations or power, see Lukes, *Power*, 1986.

scholarly focus on women's formal organizations as the site of protest against gender-based inequalities. Low-income, largely illiterate women, who constitute the majority of women in the world, have neither the time nor the skills to engage in organized formal women's organizations, and rarely do. Their voices of protest, their daily struggles and strategies, essential building blocks for the work of formal women's groups, are thus rarely known and even more rarely inform our theories of power.

However, gender-based conflict has not been part of the on-going debates on 'every day' resistance. This is partly due to the influence of the concept of "patriarchy," as developed in the feminist discourses of the 1960s and early 1970s, on shaping much of the thinking about gender.[3] The concept has been used as a blanket term to emphasize the essence and existence of one universal patriarchal system and "failed to convey movement, the complexities of relations between men and women, or the extent of women's resistance to and transformation of male power" (Ramazanoglu 1989: 38). Patriarchy was viewed as a universal, static system and a formidable power structure, with little potential to challenge except through organized international 'sisterhood' movements.

Several scholars, however, have more recently challenged this universal, essentialist, and stagnant notion of patriarchy (see Rowbotham 1981; Ramazanoglu 1989; Kandiyoti 1988), as well as its utility for identifying and understanding the specific forms of women's subordination cross-culturally. It is now well accepted that gender is constructed simultaneously with a range of other positionalities, such as class, age, and ethnicity, which thus modify, shape, and affect both women's 'gender interests' as well as their perceptions of particular social arrangements (Beneria 1992).

One of the few attempts to explicitly apply the concept of everyday resistance to gender issues is provided by Judith Okely. She argues that to capture women's subordination, we need to look beyond sustained collective action and explore the fragmented, less visible, and often isolated 'moments' of defiance and resistance located in individuals at distinct moments of their life. "Putting up a fight, i.e., not being submissive, could be interpreted as a momentary resistance to women's fundamental subordination" (Okely 1991: 7).

---

3. For an overview of the concept of patriarchy and its use by different strands of feminism, see Beechey, "On Patriarchy," *Feminist Review* 3: 66–83, 1979.

There are several reasons why women's resistance to gender-based discrimination is likely to be diffuse, non-confrontational, and subtle. The first is the powerful and mutually reinforcing relationship between gender and kinship, and between gender ideology and kinship ideology.[4] Women and men are not only females and males, but they are also mothers and fathers, wives and husbands, nieces and nephews, cousins, etc. Both in the family and in the workplace, women are enmeshed in a complex web, not only of exploitative relations, but also relations of solidarity and reciprocity, based on kinship (Joseph 1978; White 1994). Closely related is the corporate orientation that is valued in many parts of the non-western world. Women and men, do not always define themselves as individuals with separate rights independent of a larger group, but rather see themselves as part and extensions of significant others (Joseph 1993).

Moreover, women's power and status in the family in many parts of the world is often of a cyclical nature. Older women, particularly mothers-in-law, have both more autonomy as well as more power over younger women in the household (Mernissi 1975; Rassam 1980). Such a context creates conflict between women and results in a situation where women are subordinate to both men and women. Moreover, younger women can anticipate more power and authority as they go through the course of their lives, thus encouraging women's own internationalization of their subordination and undermining their need to directly challenge existing power structures (Kandiyoti 1988).

In addition, women's unequal positions are a result not only of gender, but of their structural position in the household, their class location, and national and international policies. Thus while women may be aware of the constraints under which they operate, the underlying causes of these constraints are more elusive (Macleod 1986, 1992a, 1992b). The subtle, overlapping, and diffuse nature of the constraints on women, the intermeshing of exploitation and reciprocity, and the lack of a clear person, group, or class to confront, would arguably lead to diffuse, non con-frontational, and non-coordinated forms of resistance, both in action and in expression. Several researches have, implicitly or explicitly, adopted this approach to resistance (Dwyer 1978; Rosen 1984; Abu Lughod 1986; Messik 1987; Macleod 1992; Boddy 1994).

Studies of gender relations based on a resistance framework, however, pose specific challenges. The ties between men and women are of a specific

---

4. Collier and Yanagisako, 1987, provide an excellent analysis of kinship and gender as mutually reinforcing social categories.

type. Unlike other 'subordinate' and 'dominant' groups, whose universes may only occasionally overlap, men and women usually operate within the same universe, within the same cultural text. More theoretical work, grounded in everyday lived realities, is thus required to develop new concepts that can capture the specific nature of power underlying gender relations. Women's resistance needs to be viewed as a broad continuum of immediate-, short-, medium-, and long-term strategies, which may include both passive and active forms of protest, and various stages and types of 'consciousness.' It is also essential for any study of women's resistance to identify and be particularly sensitive to the categories, interpretations, and the cultural idioms that women and men in a particular setting are themselves using to denote notions like conflict, domination, agency, etc. Researchers will have to "look beyond formal institutions and statements and into the textures of the everyday" (Comaroff 1987: 192).

Spirit Possession in Low-income Cairo

It is precisely my venture into the textures of women's everyday life in low-income Cairo that has brought spirit possession to my attention. Spirit possession in Egypt is a predominantly female phenomenon. Its belief systems and rituals were probably introduced into upper class Egypt by African slaves in the eighteenth and nineteenth centuries (Fakhouri 1968, Nelson 1971), and gradually diffused into the rest of society where they were incorporated into existing beliefs and practices. The increasing revival of 'Islamic' discourse in Egypt on the one hand, and the dismissal and ridicule of spirit possession by government officials, the media, and professionals on the other, makes women's public admission of possession to outsiders rare. Nonetheless, there are indications that spirit possession practices and beliefs are still pervasive, even among the upper class, if one is to follow the popular press.

The basic components of spirit possession and rituals as embodied in the *zar* cult have been partly described elsewhere (Kennedy 1978; Fakhouri 1968; Nelson 1971; Kenyon 1991). Briefly, a possessed woman is referred to as touched (*milammisa*), possessed (*'aleha rih*), spirit (*ginn*), or masters (*asyad*).

The spirits are both male and female and have different names, personalities, and nationalities. Anyone can get possessed, but there are some personal qualities, like vanity, *'ayaqa*, and certain actions, like pouring hot water in a toilet or going to bed crying, that may make one more vulnerable.

Possession is manifested in a range of symptoms, the most common of which are debilitating headaches, fatigue, irritability, feelings of suffocation, paralysis, and obsessions. The spirits, depending on who they are, make both material and non-material demands on the afflicted person. Once afflicted, it is very difficult to get the spirit out, they can only be appeased or placated through giving in to their demands and through participation in a special ceremony, referred to as *zar* or *hadra*. Attempts to exorcise the spirits through reading the Qur'an in the ear of the possessed by specialized sheikhs, a process called *ta'zim*, is an apparently increasing phenomena.

There are two types of spirit-appeasing ceremonies, a public one referred to as *hadra*, and a private one referred to as *zar*. The private one, commissioned by one woman in her home, seems to be on the decline because it is much more costly, and is being replaced instead by public *hadras*, which are open to anyone. A *hadra* ceremony is a heavily ritualized event orchestrated by a specialized broker, usually an older woman, called a *kudya*, and takes place in her house. Public *hadras* are held on a weekly basis. There are usually twenty to forty women at any one time, sitting on the floor, exchanging experiences and narratives of possession, and sometimes also smoking and drinking tea. Most of them come from different quarters in the city. A band of usually male musicians with drums, flutes, and tambourines play the different *daqqas* (songs/beats) associated with the different spirits. The beats range from somber ones to very joyful and festive ones. Each woman, according to the spirit(s) possessing her, has a special beat(s) to which she gets up and dances (*tifaqqar*) often with some cajoling from the lead musician. As the rhythm of the music picks up, some women go into a trance, from which they are revived through assistance from one of the other women by light strikes on their legs or back. The main objective of the ritual is to appease and satisfy the spirits so that they do not cause the symptoms from which possessed women are suffering. Not all the women who are at a *hadra* are possessed, however. Some go in an attempt to find out if they are possessed, which is revealed if they find themselves unable to resist dancing to a certain *daqqa*. This serves as a diagnostic procedure. Other women go out of curiosity, or for entertainment (*farfasha*).

Possessed women in Egypt are dismissed by middle-class professionals and by male-dominated institutions as psychotic or ignorant. Social anthropologists, however, have emphasized the importance of understanding spirit possession as a culturally meaningful act. Two general approaches have characterized the anthropological study of spirit possession. Although both have linked it to asymmetrical power relations, there are important differences between them. The first and predominant one has adopted a more functional approach, which argued that possession beliefs are a traditional means by women, and other deprived groups, for temporarily alleviating their subordinate status and a culturally sanctioned niche for momentarily stepping out of prescribed roles. The underlying assumption was one of therapy and catharsis. (Lewis 1991; Kennedy 1967; Morsy 1978). The second approach questions the potential of a functionalist view for fully appreciating a complex and multifaceted phenomena such as spirit possession. Arguing for moving the debate beyond the culturally sanctioned function of spirit possession rituals, several scholars have emphasized the need to pay closer attention to the subtle messages and views inherent in the narratives and episodes of possession.

This paper adopts the latter approach. The phenomena of spirit possession cannot be explained away as a traditional 'outlet' or 'therapy' for deprived and powerless women. It is true that possession by alien spirits enables women to make demands that temporarily step out of their prescribed roles as mothers, wives, and home mangers. However, spirit possession is best understood as representing an alternative female "world view" (Nelson 1971), an indigenous "feminist discourse" (Boddy 1995) that enables women to engage in a "complex negotiation of reality" (Crapanzo 1977). Negotiation through spirit possession is possible, because while low-income men, on the whole, tend to be skeptical of possession, they do not totally dismiss it as heresy or ignorance.

As a discourse, spirit possession provides a meaningful account of women's subordinate place in a world of transition. It is a dynamic discourse, whose text is closely related to a changing context. Like other cultural forms, spirit-possession episodes and imagery acquire new meanings and address new experiences as social relations and social boundaries are redefined during periods of change and transition (Ong 1987). The changing imagery and character of the spirits echoes changes in the broader socioeconomic and political fabric of society. Women interpret and incorporate new circumstances in the wider society into their possession beliefs and rituals (Nelson 1971).

My data support the view that spirit possession is a pervasive and potent discourse among women in low-income Cairo for the expression of unconventional views on often taboo subjects (Boddy 1990). In doing so, women are simultaneously constructing awareness of themselves and of men. Spirit possession is a potentially subservient cultural text that gives voice to women and allows them to subtly express a range of thoughts about their lives in general, and gender relations in particular, that they may not otherwise be able to overtly articulate. During both the *hadra*, and at other times, when the spirits are manifest (*zahir*), women are able to make suggestions, challenge role expectations, and express sentiments, that in an everyday context may be inadmissible. Non-possessed women, who are important audiences in such settings, can contemplate these issues and possibly pursue suggested trains of thought.

In addition to providing an alternate 'language,' spirit possession ceremonies also provide an important network for low-income Cairene women. Spirit possession ceremonies are culturally defined as separate and autonomous female space, and participation in them cements women's awareness of themselves *as* women. The *zar* and *hadra* ceremonies provide one of the few non-kin-, non-geographically based female networks in low-income Cairo, thus carving out an important and separate physical and social space for women, where they can forge new relationships outside of the confines of their daily lives. The *hadra* is female dominated and led, managed, and to a large extent 'owned' by women. Many women go to the hadras on a regular basis and a familiarity quickly develops among the 'regulars.' Some of these relationships are continued and developed outside the context and physical confines of the *hadra*.

As a discourse of defiance, there are interesting similarities between spirit-possession narratives and poetry. Lila Abu-Lugod, in her study of a small Bedouin community in Egypt, shows how *ghiniwas*, short poems similar to "Japanese haiku in form but more like American blues in content and emotional tone," and sung largely by women and only among them, express personal sentiments of love, loss, vulnerability, and a wide range of other interpersonal relations that go against the prevalent code of honor. Poetry among Bedouin women is a particular form of women's discourse that complements the more formal and visible discourse on gender relations. Abu Lughod concludes that "poetry as a discourse of defiance of the system symbolizes freedom" and "provides a corrective to an obsession with morality and an overzealous adherence to the ideology of honor and maybe the vision is cherished because people sense that the costs of this system of honor ideology, in the limits it places on human experience is just too high" (Abu Lughod 1987: 258–59). Spirit possession may be understood in the same light. Spirit possession narratives, like *ghiniwas*, represent not only complementary discourse, but also a culturally legitimate and 'honorable' way for women to communicate 'immodest sentiments.'

Boddy's work on spirit possession, based on fieldwork in a village in the Sudan, is perhaps the best illustration of possession as a discourse of resistance. Focusing on the 'articulatory potential' of possession, she argues that signals and messages women deduce from their own possession and from observing the episodes of possession in other women defies, challenges, and reworks conventional meanings of gender relations, opening up provocative, albeit ambiguous and opaque, directions of thought. "Messages communicated by women to both male and female villagers via the *zar* often have subversive tones as well as supportive ones. Gender-appropriate meanings emerge when individuals read these messages in light of their own experiences. Boddy concludes, "possession can thus amplify a woman's double consciousness to the point where she is able to see her life, her society, her sender, from an altered perspective and a heightened sense of awareness" (Boddy 1989: 5). In the following section, I want to illustrate how the discourse of possession enables low-income women in Cairo to comment on and challenge dominant gender discourses by looking at recurring messages that emerged from my interviews and discussions.

Religion and Sex: Voices that Refuse to be Silenced

The data presented below are based on in-depth interviews with twelve possessed women and their families in a 'low-income' community on the outskirts of Cairo, and eleven visits to public spirit-possession ceremonies in three other low-income quarters. All the interviewees were Muslim women, and the majority, married and illiterate. Three women, however, held a technical high-school-level diploma, and three were single. All interviews were taped. During my interviews and observations, I was most interested in listening closely to what possessed women were saying about their lives, to what the spirits, when manifest, were saying, and to what specific demands they made on the women. Two themes of relevance to the construction of gender relations recurred in my interviews and discussions: religion and sex.

One of the first observations that struck me was that most of the women I talked to were possessed by Christian spirits.[5] I had not seen

---

5. In her study of a spirit possession/healing cult in the Sudan, Kenyon does make reference to the *khawajat* (foreigners) as an important category in the *tombura zar*, but she does not elaborate on the significance of foreign, presumably Christian, spirits operating in a predominantly Muslim context

reference to this tendency in the literature and I was quite puzzled. During the hadras I attended, the one beat that was repeated the most and to which people danced—*faqqaru*—was the monastery beat *(daqqat al-der)*, which is requested by Christian spirits. Christian spirits, referred to by women as misihiyin, made a series of demands on the women. These included purchasing silver pendants with a cross and Christ on them, going to church, drinking beer, refusing to pray according to Islamic precepts, and refusing to wear the veil. The women possessed by Christian spirits could not stand to hear the Qur'an and the call for prayer, or to pray themselves.

I am possessed by two *misihi ginn*, Girgis and Mary. My beat is the monastery beat *(daqqat al-der)*. I just find myself pulled when I hear it and I keep dancing. But I also like to dance to the beat of the Prophet *(madih al-nabi)*. Mary and Girgis are young and they want me to wear short skirts and trousers and not to pray. When I hear the call to prayer I keep screaming and have to close my ears. I want to wear the veil, but they do not allow me. I tried once and I had a continuous headache for two weeks. I had to stay in a dark room and tie my head from the pain. My mother took me to many doctors but nothing worked. (Sanaa, a 19-year-old woman finishing her diploma in nursing)

I know I am possessed by a Christian spirit because I saw him several years ago. I still feel him sleeping beside me when I go to bed. He is a priest, and he is tall, white, and good-looking. He asked me to buy a silver cross and I got one and have been wearing it ever since. I have always prayed regularly and read the Qur'an, but he does not like it. Now, when I pray, I feel like someone is choking me and I fall down. (Umm Samya, a 40-year-old married woman with two daughters)

I stopped praying and insisted on buying a dog. People told me this was bad because a dog in a house makes the angels go away. But I was very attached to this dog. I used to walk like a madwoman in the street and then suddenly I would fall down unconscious in the form of a cross *(atsalib)*. I went to many doctors, but they could not heal me. My neighbor suggested that I go and have my *qatar* seen, and I did. [Qatar is an item of clothing or scent used to diagnose spirit afflictions.] The *kudya* told me that I am possessed by a Christian spirit who is in love with me and wants me to make him a *zar*. I made him a *zar* and I got all the things that Christian spirits like, you know they are like foreigners *(khawagat)*. I had a large buffet with Greek cheese *(gibna rumi)*, olives, and beer. I invited many friends. I felt much better afterward, but every now and then the symptoms come back. . . . Just last week my daughters found me tearing my clothes as a taped recitation of the Qur'an was on. (Umm Neamat, married with two daughters)

I asked women why so many of the spirits were Christian, and whether this was a new phenomenon. One of my interviewees, an elder woman who has been possessed for many years, explained that there are many more Christian spirits nowadays than in the past. I heard that this is because the priest in the nearby community, Father Sam'an, has asked the Christian spirits to spread to our community *(sarahhum 'alena)*. Another woman ventured a similar conspiracy interpretation, but at a more global level: "It is because the grand pope in America, the head of the Christians, has asked the spirits to go to the Muslim world and possess Muslim women. They want us to be Christian *(nasara)* like them."

Amal, a married woman who has been possessed by two Christian spirits for the past years had a different interpretation: "The spirits are not really Christian. They are all Muslim and they are good. We just say they are Christian because Christian spirits are stronger, they are more difficult to get out when the sheikhs come and read Qur'an *(ya'azimo)*. Muslim spirits may respond to the sheikhs' use of Qur'an but Christian ones do not, and so the Qur'an cannot get them out. The most that a sheikh can do is to make them become Muslims." I was told of several cases when a sheikh could not get the spirit out, but at least managed to convert them to Islam. According to the women I interviewed, however, the resort to sheikhs to get the spirits out, and the attempt to convert the spirits is a phenomenon that has become widespread only in the past seven or eight years.

The above illustrations provide a provocative commentary by women on their lives. They also suggest that the imagery of the spirits is closely related to specific socioeconomic and political contexts. The fact that so many spirits are Christians and their specific 'anti-Islamic' demands could also be a reflection of the increasing intrusion of 'Islam' into these women's life and the increasing pressure from community leaders and the media on women to display more obvious Islamic behavior. Formal Islamic discourse is against *zars*. Possessed women are considered weak in faith *(imanhum da'if)*. They are under tremendous pressure by local religious leaders and authorities to become more pious, to take the veil, to pray, and to read the Qur'an regularly. In such a context, spirit possession offers a 'counter-hegemonic' discourse. Women's resistance to such an increasingly 'Islamic' public discourse, or at least their perception that such a discourse can undermine their status or threaten them, may be reflected in an increase in possession by Christian spirits.

The other theme that emerged from my interviews relates to sex. Sexuality is a critical component in the construction of gender relations in the Middle East. Sawsan Al Messiri (1978) notes that men's ability to keep their wives sexually satisfied through "frequent and lengthy intercourse" is an essential element of both men's and women's notions of masculinity in low-income *(baladi)* Cairo. Moreover, a local urban woman *(bint al-balad)* is very aware of herself as a sexual, feminine being and this self-image is reflected in the seductive way she wraps her traditional cover *(milaya laff)* around her hips and in her coquettish walk. Insights into the importance of sexuality in the construction of gender identities can also be gleaned from Lawrence Rosen's (1978) study in the city of Serou, Morocco. His research revealed that men differentiated themselves from women on the basis of fundamental differences in sexual nature. Women are viewed by men to possess much more *nifs*—the thoughts and attributes such as lust and passion that people have in common with animals—than *'aql*—reason and rationality. Rosen's male informants argued that women's excessive sexual desire is the reason they are locally referred to as 'the rope of Satan' *(habl al-shitan)* and necessitates that men, whom nature has equipped with much more *'aql*, systematically control women. The Moroccan woman, described by one of Rosen's informants, is "like a Turkish bath without water, because she is always hot and without a man she has no way to slake the fire" (Rosen 1978: 567).

What was interesting to me is that women's commentary about their sexual relationships revealed through possession narratives differed from the above descriptions. The women I interviewed expressed not excessive desire, but a consistent lack of sexual desire or sexual interest, at least in the context of their marital relations. The following excerpts from interviews illustrate the opaque, ambiguous, but also challenging, commentary of women on their sexual lives.

> I have not been sleeping in the same bed with my husband for the past ten years and we have not had sex for that long. There is nothing I can do about it. The spirits do not allow me. When he comes near me I start kicking and screaming. One day I bit him so hard he bled. At first my husband used to get angry and hit me, but now he understands that it is not up to me. The masters (*asyad*) do not want it. I know it is forbidden (*haram*) to deny my husband sex, and I have been to many doctors and I even made a *zar* every year for the past three years, but the spirits still do not allow me; it is out of my control. I personally do not mind it however. I never enjoyed sex with him. It was always a duty. Sometimes he also hurts me. (Umm Yusif, a married woman with three children)

> He is a stupid ox (*'igl*) and I despise him. He is trying to sleep with me and is asking me to do dirty things (*hagat wiskha*). I love Amal (Umm Ayman) and I do not want her to sleep with him, so every time he tries to sleep with her, I get in the middle of the bed and separate them and kick him. So one day, he said, 'Fine. If Amal does not want to sleep with me, then you sleep with me.' I am a man like him, but he is not ashamed to ask me to do these things. He is a very bad man. ('Abdallah, a spirit possessing Umm Ayman and speaking to the author when he was manifest during one my interviews. He spoke through Umm Ayman, but in an altered voice.)

> Mukhlis, the spirit, has been with me for three years, before I got married, but I did not know it then. He made me refuse all marriage proposals. I got married in the end because Mukhlis succumbed and let me get married. My eldest brother—I am the only girl among three bothers—insisted that I marry and beat me up for refusing. Mukhlis did not want to see me beaten up so in the end he agreed and I got married to my current husband. Since I

got married, however, I have had terrible headaches. I also hate sleeping with my husband. When he approaches me I start screaming and I feel as if someone is strangling me. Mukhlis manifested himself to me at a friend's *zar* that I attended six months ago. He manifested himself as a tall pink-skinned giant with dark black hair. He told me he was in love with me and explained that he makes sex unbearable with my husband because he is jealous. Now I sometimes see Mukhlis sleeping beside me on the bed, and I can feel his breath on my neck. (Amal, a married woman with two small children)

I get pain *(batwagga')* when I sleep with my husband. I do not enjoy it *(mafish inbisat)*. I just wait for it to end. I am cold *(barda)*. Samar told me that she had a similar situation and that someone advised her to see her '*attar*. She discovered that she was possessed by Yawer Bey. He is a very snobbish man and he hurts her when she has sex with her husband because he does not like her husband. You see her husband is not a respectable man. He does not give her enough money to buy proper clothes or household items, even though he earns a lot. Samar suggested that maybe I am also possessed. Maybe the spirit is angry with my husband too. He also does not provide for me. I will go with her to a *hadra* this week. (Umm Yusif, a newly married woman)

What messages can one derive from such comments? What does it tell us and women in the community about how women view their own sexuality, their sexual relations with their husbands, their role as sexual partners, and the extent to which they have control over sexual circumstances, i.e., when, with whom, and how to have sex, particularly in a context where refusing sex is considered a religious sin *(haram)*? While the messages are not clear and can be interpreted differently by different women, several suggestions can be teased out: women do not enjoy sex with their husbands, their husbands do not satisfy them sexually, their husbands request "improper" sexual demands, women's sexual submission is linked to men's ability to provide for them. The list can go on. One striking aspect is the intimate language in which women talk about the spirits, not as intruders, but as protectors and sometimes lovers. The important point to note here, however, is that such comments suggest that women have developed a 'hidden transcript,' that is, a set of meanings shared in separate circles away from and beyond the domination of public and male fora (Scott 1990). This discourse is a result of, and contributes to women's self-awareness and consciousness of gender-based power. Its contradictory and ambivalent messages are partly what enable it to prevail.

The Limitations of the 'Hidden Transcript'

In the search for the 'infra-politics' of subordinate groups, there is a danger of romanticizing resistance. By romanticizing, I mean reading all forms of everyday resistance, and potential resistance, as signs of the ineffectiveness of systems of power and a celebration of the resilience, creativity, and free spirit of human beings in their refusal to accept oppression (O'Hanlon 1991; Abu-Lughod 1990). Particularly as used in the early work of James Scott, the concept of every day forms of resistance does not fully appreciate the cultural and ideological aspects of domination and the structural constraints which limit the actions of subordinate groups, and lay down distinct 'rules of the game,' which largely determine what they can resist and how effective they can be. There is a danger of overemphasizing the ability of subordinate groups to always penetrate the hegemonic ideologies of the ruling classes and to develop a free discourse and consciousness. As D. Haynes and G. Prakash (1991) have correctly argued, the ability of subordinate groups to break through the walls of hegemony is constrained by the very nature of existing power structures; every day acts of resistance take place in the field of power and thus are themselves affected by the nature of hegemony.

While my data support the view that the idiom of possession can indeed be a powerful 'hidden transcript' for women, a cover language of protest that enables them to comment on, and contemplate their self awareness as women, such a discourse does not escape the categories of formal dominant discourses and is limited by them. The danger of romanticizing every day forms to resistance, in this case spirit possession, is well illustrated by an inadequately publicized murder case published in *al-Ahram* in June 1995 under the headline, "Possessed girl beaten to death by her father to get the spirits out of her body." On June 3, 1995, Sahar Emad Eddin Yousser, a 13-year-old girl who lives in Mansura was found dead in her room. The cause of death was repeated beatings with a plastic hose. Investigations revealed that the girl's parents, both engineers had taken up the 'Islamic dress' last year, quit their work, and started pressuring their daughter to take up the veil. She refused, apparently because she is possessed and the spirits are not allowing her to take the veil. After several months of pressuring her, her parents kept her from school, locked her in a room, and started beating her with a plastic hose to get the spirits out. Sahar's spirits of resistance were defeated. She died. What messages members of her community derived from this episode is difficult to judge.

Conclusions

In this paper I have pursued the argument that spirit possession among low-income women can best be understood as an expressive form. Spirit possession ceremonies, episodes, rituals, and narratives offer an arena for the emergence of women's unofficial world views, their 'hidden transcripts,' and creates a platform for the articulation of dissatisfaction and of provocative and defiant ideas and sentiments on a range of issues that in normal every day discourse would be unacceptable or dangerous to reveal. An examination of women's narratives of possession reveals a rich, unconventional, yet subtle and ambiguous commentary on their lives and their relationships with men and the wider society. I have attempted to illustrate this argument by focusing on two themes that have emerged from my interviews with possessed women: sexual relations and religion. While potentially powerful and provocative, however, I have also argued that spirit possession as a discourse of defiance is not completely liberating. Because it operates within the framework of dominant structures and discourses, its impact on challenging power relations has inherent limitations, and its maintenance often comes at a tremendous cost, emotionally, and, as the example of Sahar illustrates, possibly physically as well.

One of the important issues that emerges from the fieldwork also relates to the relationship between 'formal' Islamic discourses as dominant and male-centric ideologies, and spirit possession as a predominantly female belief system. The relationship is a complex and increasingly tense one, and this is partly reflected in the images and demands of the spirits. Women, however are careful to give a religious basis to their own activities and beliefs. They are continuously attempting to normalize spirit possession and its rituals through invoking the Qur'an and Islamic terms. On the other hand, formal Islamic discourse is increasingly contesting these practices and targeting possessed women in an attempt to marginalize them and their rituals. At a national level, such attempts are clear in the recent Egyptian commercial films, such as the 1990 film al-*Bayda wa-l-hagara* (The Egg and the Stone) directed by 'Ali 'Abdel Khaleq, which depict possession and its rituals as a form of moral decadence and a facade for illegal activities such as prostitution and drug dealing, depictions strongly abhorred and denied by all the women I interviewed, and of which I saw no indication during my over 11 visits to different hadras. The apparently recent processes of *ta'zim*, and attempts at spirit conversion mentioned earlier, are also striking examples of the extent to which spirit possession beliefs are being targeted at the local, community level. There appears to be a fair degree of resistance on the part of women, however, to hold on to spirit possession, which is reflected both in using the same dominant discourse to justify their actions, but also possibly through the unconscious or conscious manipulation of the imagery and demands of the spirits. Although a study like this one cannot talk with any authority about trends over time, many of my interviewees stressed that they know more possessed women now than in the past, and that while the incidence of the *zar*, as the more elaborate, private ceremony, has decreased, the *hadras* are still a resilient and important feature of low-income women's lives. What is important stress is that the importance of *hadras* goes beyond the numbers of women who are possessed or who physically attend them, to the many other women who are directly or indirectly affected by the larger discourse of spirit possession.

Bibliography

Abu Lughod, Lila, 1990, "The Romance of Resistance: Tracing Transformations of Power through Bedouin Women," *American Ethnologist*, 17: 41–55.

———, 1986, *Veiled Sentiments: Honor and Poetry in a Bedouin Society*. Berkeley and Los Angeles: University of California Press.

Beechey, Veronica. 1979, "On patriarchy," *Feminist Review*, 3: 66–82.

Beneria, L., 1992, "Accounting for Women's Work: The Progress of Two Decades," *World Development*, 20 (11): 1547–1560.

Boddy, Janice Patricia, 1994, "Spirit Possession Revisited: Beyond Instrumentality," *Annual Review of Anthropology*, 23: 407–434.

———, 1989, *Wombs and Alien Spirits: Women, Men, and the Zar Cult in Northern Sudan*. Madison: University of Wisconsin Press.

Comaroff, J. and Jean Comaroff, 1987, "The Madman and the Migrant: Work and Labor in the Historical Consciousness of a South African People," *American Ethnologist*, 14 (2), 191–209.

Crapanzano, Vincent, 1977, *In Case Studies of Possession*. Vincent Crapanzano and Vivian Garrison, eds. New York: John Wiley.

Dwyer, Daisy, 1978, *Images and Self Images: Male and Female in Morocco*. New York: Columbia University Press.

Fakhouri, Hani, 1968, "The Zar Cult in an Egyptian Village," *Anthropological Quarterly*, 41 (2): 49–77.

Foucault, Michel, 1986, "Disciplinary Power and Subjection," *Power*. Steven Lukes, ed. Oxford: Basil Blackwell.

————, 1981, *History of Sexuality: An Introduction*, vol. 1. New York: Random House.

Gramsci, Antonio, 1995, *Further Selections from the Prison Notebooks*, Derek Boothman, ed. Minneapolis: University of Minnesota Press.

Haynes, D. and G. Prakash, eds., 1991, *Contesting Power: Resistance and Everyday Social Relations in South Asia*. Delhi: Oxford University Press.

Hoare, Quinton and Geoffry Nowell Smith, eds., 1971, *Antonio Gramasci: Selections from the Prison Notebooks*. New York: International Publishers.

Holub, Renate, 1992, *Antonio Gramsci: Beyond Marxism and Post Modernism*. London: Routledge.

Joseph, Suad, 1999, *Intimate Selving in Arab Families: Gender, Self, and Identity*. Syracuse: Syracuse University Press.

————, 1993, "Gender and Relationality among Arab Families In Lebanon," *Feminist Studies*, 19 (3): 465–486.

————, 1978, "Women and the Neighborhood Street in Borj Hammoud, Lebanon," *Women in the Muslim World*, N. Keddie and L. Beck, eds. Cambridge: Harvard University Press.

Kandiyoti, Deniz, 1998, "Gender, Power, and Contestation: Rethinking Bargaining with Patriarchy," *Divided We Stand: Gender Analysis and Development Issues*, R. Pearson and C. Sacks, eds. London: Routledge.

————, 1988, "Bargaining with Patriarchy," *Gender and Society*, 2 (3): 274–290.

Kennedy, John, 1967, "Nubian Zar Ceremonies as Psychotherapy," *Human Organisation*, 26 (4): 186–194.

Kenyon, Susan, 1991, *Five Women of Sennar: Culture and Change in Central Sudan*. Oxford: Clarendon Press.

Lewis, I.M., A. Al-Safi, and S. Hurreiz, 1991, *Women's Medicine: The Zar Bori Cult in Africa and Beyond*. Edinburgh: Edinburgh University Press for the International African Institute.

Lukes, Steven, 1986, *Power*. Oxford: Basil Blackwell.

MacLeod, Arlene, E., 1992, "Hegemonic Relations and Gender Resistance: The New Veiling as Accommodating Protest in Cairo," *Signs: Journal of Women in Culture and Society*, 17 (31): 533–557.

———, 1992a, "Hegemonic Relations and Gender Resistance: The New Veiling as Accommodating Protest in Cairo," *Signs: Journal of Women in Culture and Society*, 17(31): 533–557.

———, 1992b, *Accommodating Protest: Working Women, the New Veiling, and Change in Cairo*. Cairo: The American University in Cairo Press.

———, 1986, *Hegemony and Women: Working and Re-veiling in Cairo, Egypt*. Paper presented at the Northeastern Political Science Association Annual Meeting, November.

McLellan, David, 1973, *Karl Marx: His Life and Thought*. London: Macmillan Press.

McNay, Lois, 1992, *Foucault and Feminism*. Cambridge: Polity Press.

Mernissi, Fatima, 1975, *Beyond the Veil: Male-Female Dynamics in a Modern Muslim Society*. New York: John Wiley and Sons.

Messick, Brinkley, 1987, "Subordinate Discourse: Women, Weaving, and Gender Relations in North Africa," *American Ethnologist*, 14 (2): 210–25

Al-Messiri, Sawsan, 1978, "Self Images of Traditional Urban Women in Cairo," *Women in the Muslim World*, Beck. L. and N. Keddi, eds. Cambridge: Harvard University Press.

Morsy, Soheir, 1978, "Sex Differences and Folk Illness in an Egyptian Village," *Women in the Muslim World*, op. cit.

Nelson, Cynthia, 1971, "Self, Spirit Possession, and World View: An illustration from Egypt," *International Journal of Social Psychiatry*, 17: 194–209.

O'Hanlon, Rosalind, 1991, "Issues of Widowhood: Gender and Resistance in Colonial Western India," *Contesting Power: Resistance and Everyday Social Relations in South Asia*, D. Haynes and G. Prakash, eds. Delhi: Oxford University Press.

———, 1988, "Recovering the Subject: Subaltern Studies and Histories of Resistance in Colonial South Asia," *Modern Asian Studies*, 22 (1): 189–224.

Okely, Judith, 1991, "Defiant Moments: Gender, Resistance, and Individuals," *Man*, 26: 189–224.

Ong, Ahiwa, 1987, *Spirits of Resistance and Capitalist Discipline: Factory Women in Malaysia*. New York: State University of New York Press.

Ramazanoglu, Caroline, 1989, *Feminism and the Contradictions of Oppression*. London: Routledge.

———, 1999, *Feminism and the Contradictions of Oppression*. London: Routledge.

Rassam, Amal, 1980, "Women and Domestic Power in Morocco," *International Journal of Middle East Studies*, 12: 171–179.

Raymond Williams, 1977, *Marxism and Literature*. London: Oxford University Press.

Rosen, Lawrence, 1984, *The Anthropology of Justice: Law as Culture in Islamic Society*. Cambridge: Cambridge University Press.

Rosen, Lawrence, 1978, "The Negotiation of Reality: Male and Female Relations in Sefrou, Morocco," *Women in the Muslim World*, op. cit.

Rowbotham, S., 1981, "The Trouble with Patriarchy," *People's History and Socialist Theory*, R. Samuel, ed. London: Routledge and Kegan.

Scott, James, 1990, *Domination and the Arts of Resistance: Hidden Transcripts*. New Haven: Yale University Press.

———, 1986, "Everyday Forms of Resistance," *Journal of Peasant Studies*, 13 (2): 5–35.

———, 1985, *Weapons of the Weak: Every Days Forms of Resistance*. New Haven: Yale University Press, 1985.

Strathern, M., 1987, "An Awkward Relationship: The Case of Feminism and Anthropology," *Signs: Journal of Women in Culture and Society*, 2 (21): 276–292.

Turton, Andrew, 1986, "Patrolling the Middle Ground: Methodological Perspectives on 'Everyday Peasant Resistance,'" *Journal of Peasant Studies*, 13 (2): 36–48.

White, Christine Pelzer, 1986, "Everyday Resistance, Socialist Revolution, and Rural Development: The Vietnamese Case," Journal of Peasant Studies, 13 (2): 49–63.

White, Jenny. B. 1994. *Money Makes Us Relatives: Women's Labor in Urban Turkey*. Austin: University of Texas Press.

Quest for Beauty

Globalization, Identity, and the Production of Gendered Bodies in Low-income Cairo

FARHA GHANNAM

The body is very much in the news in Egypt and other parts of the Middle East. Organ transplants, cloning, abortion, circumcision, and, lately, weight loss have become parts of public debates in Egyptian media, mosques, and schools. Weight loss in particular has been discussed in local and international newspapers. Recently, the *Wall Street Journal* (March 4, 1998) reported that there is a growing concern over weight in Egypt as manifested in the proliferation of support groups, dietary information, fitness centers, and weight-loss clinics in Cairo. The newspaper interviewed an Egyptian woman, Samia Alluba, who has been trying to promote exercise and fitness. She was happy because her "work is beginning to pay off." "Slimness," she declares, is increasingly perceived "as something beautiful." What attracted the attention of the reporter was the newness of this phenomenon and the fact that "[t]he head of Egyptian television recently announced that overweight female newscasters (more than twenty) have three months to shed those extra pounds (10 to 20 pounds in most cases) or they will be fired." Farida El-Zommor, a prominent Egyptian broadcaster, argued that the decision was unfair. She stated that "all Egyptian women are overweight," that it is "inevitable" to gain weight in Cairo, and that "losing weight is practically un-Egyptian." After explaining how difficult it is to walk in Cairo and to secure money for exercising and dieting, El-Zommor supported her argument by saying, "Look at Oprah Winfrey. She is a talented television personality, and she is fat." When the reporter told her that Oprah had lost weight, El-Zommor argued that "[s]he must not be too beautiful anymore then."

The competing ideals of the body expressed in the interviews with El-Zommor (preference for the plump body) and Alluba (thinness is beautiful) are part of wider struggles taking place in various classes and areas in Egypt.[1] Drawing on my study in a low-income neighborhood in northern Cairo (which I will call Little Cairo), during 1993–94 and 1997,[2] I argue in this chapter that globalization (i.e., the flow of information, capital, labor, goods and people between different parts of the world) facilitates the circulation of various images and products that mark new desirable forms of the body.

The television set in particular is powerful in circulating information and images about the bodily forms and stimulating desires for new products. This flow of images and a growing market of beauty products present new ideas and possibilities about the body that were not available to older women. My aim here is not to document the changes in preferences in bodily forms and images over the years, although such a documentation is very much needed. Rather, I want to look at how some competing images and desires are being negotiated by young women in the formation of their bodies and self-identification.

The following discussion focuses on how young single women (between the age of 15–25) struggle with various competing ideas about beauty and preferred bodily forms. I first provide a brief review of the body as the object of study in social sciences and then discuss how the body and its representation are central to the identity of young women. Focusing on ideals of beauty, I aim to highlight differences between women based on age, education, and access to information, and how these differences inform their efforts to shape their bodies. To illustrate this, I present a detailed case study to show how young women try to remake their bodies and how beauty is closely linked with social views and self-identity.

---

1. Recently, actress Laila Elwi became the focus of criticism in Egyptian newspapers due to her increasing weight. One writer suggested that the head of the television should interfere to stop the increase in Elwi's weight.

2. My field work during 1993–1994 was supported by the Middle East Awards (MEAwards) and the Wenner-Gren Foundation. The field research during 1997 was supported by the Reproductive Health Working Group, the Population Council. The support of these institutions is very much appreciated.

The Body as the Object of Study

In the past two decades, the body has attracted more attention and has become the center of a wide range of studies that examine the role of the body in the formation of subjects and the reproduction of social life (Foucault 1979, 1980, 1990; Bourdieu 1984, 1990; Frank 1991; Turner 1992, 1991a; Good 1994). The increasing attention to the body in the last twenty years is related to several changes (Shilling 1993; Turner 1991, 1991a; Frank 1991; Martin 1992; Synnott 1992; Grosz 1994; Gilman 1999). First, feminist struggles brought attention to many questions related to the female body such as fertility, sexuality, and gender relationships. Second, new demographic changes in the west (such as the increase in the number of the elderly) as well as the AIDS crisis and growing environmental pollution raised many policy issues such as pension and healthcare. Third, the growth of the 'consumer culture,' which highlighted awareness of physical potentials, emphasized the body as a 'machine' that could be shaped in various ways, and increased the importance of the body to the formation of self-identity. The tendency toward equating the body with self-identification has led to a growing interest in shaping, maintaining, and beautifying the body (Shilling 1993; Synnott 1993; Featherstone et al. 1991; Turner 1991a). At the same time, the increasing control over the body (mainly through medical technology), opened it for questioning and created uncertainties about the body, its 'meanings,' and 'boundaries.' (Shilling 1993; Turner 1991a; Synnott 1992; Balsamo 1996). These changes accelerated conflicts and disagreements around many issues related to the body, especially the female body, such as abortion, suicide, new reproductive technologies, and questions related to who has the right to control the body (Synnott 1993). All these changes raised theoretical and methodological questions about the study of the body, especially the gendered body, its construction, health, and identification.

A major part of the current literature focuses on exploring the impact of 'modern' techniques and how they shape perceptions of the body. This literature is based on a dichotomy between 'our' bodies that are modern (i.e., western) and 'their' bodies (i.e., non-modern, which equals non-western). This emphasis gives the impression that modern bodies are more (deliberately) socially constructed than non-modern bodies (Shilling 1993; Turner 1991a). Several authors justify this dichotomy by suggesting that while 'pre-modern' bodies were "marked by traditional signs in ritualized settings," the body in "the affluent west" is treated mainly as "a phenomenon to be shaped, decorated, and trained as an expression of an *individual's* identity" (Shilling 1993: 4, 200).[3]

This tendency is clearly manifested in the work of Pierre Bourdieu. One can distinguish 'two bodies,' so to speak, in the various studies that Bourdieu has published since the early 1960s. His work in Algeria (1977, 1990) brought into focus the body and its role in the objectification of illiterate cultures and the inscription of social inequalities on the body. In societies where education is not developed, such as Algeria in the 1960s, the body becomes the main space where the habitus (a set of internalized dispositions that structures and regulates practices) is inscribed (Bourdieu 1990, 1977). Many social inequalities are embodied, i.e., become parts of the body's appearance, movements, gestures, and usage. This embodiment situates the fundamental principles of practices below consciousness and language, which means that the habitus "cannot be touched by voluntary, deliberate transformation" (Bourdieu 1977: 94). Embodiment also reinforces beliefs in dominant "systems of classification by making it appear to be grounded in reality" in the eyes of the dominant and the dominated groups, i.e., naturalized (Bourdieu 1990: 71).

The 'Algerian body' manifests and reinforces the opposition between male and female. Gender differences are marked by walking, eating, and other daily activities. Biological differences are highlighted and symbolically emphasized by differences in movements and gestures that reveal the social position of the agent and manifest a whole relationship to the world. The habitus generates a biological interpretation of social characteristics and a social interpretation of biological features so that both of them are leading to the other and are reinforcing each other. The opposition between male and female becomes the main (and only) division that structures the constitution of "self-image and world-image" (Bourdieu 1990: 78).

In his study of classes in France (1984), Bourdieu's primary interest is the commodification of the body. He analyzes it as a physical capital that can be converted into economic, social, and cultural capital and is

---

3. Until recently, most theories of the body have focused on the history of the 'western' body and its contemporary constructions. These theories should be problematized when used in the study of the body and the self in non-western contexts. This problematization is not to reproduce the dichotomy between modern and traditional societies, but to challenge and transcend such categories and classifications, and to recognize that all bodies are socially constructed, be it in the west or the east; what should be examined is how they are constructed.

central to gaining access to material resources and achieving distinction (cultural value). The preferred bodily properties are not randomly distributed but there is a continuous struggle between classes (and their fractions) to define, appropriate, and transform the valuable forms of body to achieve distinction (Bourdieu 1984). Here, the body becomes the "most indisputable materialization of class taste" (190). Taste, "a class culture turned into nature, that is, *embodied*" shapes the "class body" (90). It "unites and separates" in the sense that it brings people who share the same taste (i.e., occupy the same social space) together (by claiming to be natural) and differentiates them from others whose taste is assumed to be unnatural (56, 190).

Orientations towards bodily features differ greatly between classes. Tastes and the selection of food depend on the perceptions of the body and the effects of food on the body's "strength, health, and beauty" (Bourdieu 1984: 190). For example, working-class people pay more attention to the strength of the male body and therefore tend to select the cheapest, most filling, and fatty meals, which secure the reproduction of the labor force at minimum cost. Professionals tend to select what is "tasty, health-giving, light, and not fattening" (190). Thus, it is possible to "map out a universe of class bodies, which (biological accidents apart) tends to reproduce in its specific logic the universe of the social structure" (193).

Unlike his sophisticated analysis of the body in France, Bourdieu's discussion of the 'Algerian body' is static and reductionist. While in France there is a continuous struggle over the body, and its meaning and signification between classes, the 'Algerian body' simply mirrors and reproduces gender inequalities. Bourdieu's model has been criticized by many scholars (such as de Certeau 1984, Harker et al 1990, Shilling 1993). A major part of the critique is centered around the unconscious nature of the habitus that Bourdieu tends to emphasize in most of his work. The over-determination that results from Bourdieu's conceptualization of the habitus makes it hard to account for agency and intentionality. Social agents are reduced to passive constrained actors with very limited choices. This over-determination also has serious implications for the theorization of social change and the possibility of challenging the status quo. Bourdieu's tendency to present the habitus as a determining force could be avoided if we use it as a "mediating construct not a determining one" (Mahar et al. 1990: 12). As Shilling emphasizes, "far from completely internalizing behavioral codes, it could be argued that individuals *selectively* apply standards depending upon the shifting contexts they inhabit" (Shilling 1993: 172).

The implications of Bourdieu's assumptions are illustrated in a more recent study by Carol Delaney of procreation in Turkey. Like Bourdieu, Delaney emphasizes the importance of the body for "illiterate villagers" because "bodies signify, they mean things" (Delaney 1991: 25). She also sees the opposition between male (the seed) and female (the soil) as structuring the relationships of the villagers with each other and with the universe. In line with Bourdieu's analysis of gender inequalities in Algeria, Delaney presents the distinction between men and women as an absolute one and pays no attention to variations within each category. There are no differences between daughters and mothers, or between sons and fathers, and no room for change based on new information or education. The village is presented as a bounded entity that is insulated from the global flow of information and images. Secular education, magazines, the village library, tape recorders, television sets (there are at least two television sets in the village tearooms), and visits to the city are not changing gender ideologies and perceptions of the body. Even though "a number of villagers remarked that when television came, the art of conversation . . . went away" (251), Delaney does not grant any power to such means in transforming and reshaping gender relationships and views of the body. She continues to emphasize that to change the place of the woman and perceptions of her role is "equivalent to unhinging the world and letting it spin off into chaos" (232). In her attempt to critique Bourdieu's limited attention to religion, Delaney goes to the other extreme in showing Islam as *the* "embracing context" for the ideas and practices of the villagers. This emphasis on Islam and the fact that she dismisses all other discourses in shaping gender relationships and procreation makes it impossible to see how things may change. She concludes that to challenge gender distinctions and to "acknowledge the equal status of men and women . . . is to rock the foundation of the universe" (225–26).

At the same time, Delaney tends to reduce the identity of a woman to her reproductive function. Fertility, as argued by several authors, is central to a woman's identity (see, for example, Inhorn 1994, 1996). But the identity of a woman cannot be reduced to this function. Fertility is only one part, albeit a very important one, of a woman's life, and her identity cannot and should not be reduced to her fertile years. In addition, the fertility of women is often taken for granted. Until the opposite has been proven, every woman is assumed to be able to have children. Thus fertility does not determine the identity of young women before marriage. Cultural and social skills, education, manners, and beauty are all central to a young woman's status and distinction.

Perhaps more than anything else, interest in beauty and bodily appearances differentiate mothers (age 45–55) from their daughters (age 15–25) in Little Cairo. Unlike their mothers who are not expected to pay much attention to their looks, especially in public, beauty is central to young women's self-identification and distinction. My argument in the rest of this chapter is directed against the tendency to view women as a unified and homogeneous group, in the process suppressing important factors such as age and education that intersect with gender in shaping self-identity. The discussion pays special attention to how young women negotiate the flow of competing discourses and images in the formation of their views of the desirable female body. In the following, I examine the body as both "product and process" (Balsamo 1996: 3). As a product, the body is the "material embodiment" of various identities and inequalities and "a staged performance of personal identity, of beauty, of health (among other things)" (3). As a process, the body is "a way of knowing and marking the world, as well as a way of knowing and making a 'self'" (3).

Like Mother, Like Daughter?
Ideals of Beauty in Little Cairo

Since the early 1960s, Little Cairo has been the home of families that migrated to the Egyptian capital from the countryside and other parts of Cairo. Its inhabitants work as petty traders, vendors, plumbers, metal and construction workers, shoemakers, factory laborers, craftsmen, mechanics, drivers, waiters, low-level government employees, teachers, and managers in small shops and businesses. There are families with relatively high income, especially those with family members who work in oil-producing countries, and there are unskilled workers with incomes that hardly sustain their families. Many men have more than one job to meet the needs of their families. Young women are usually factory workers, sales people in local shops (especially clothing), or secretaries. However, they tend to leave employment after securing enough money for their trousseau. Most stop working outside the home after marriage but many later become engaged in various economic activities around the housing unit.

In addition to more access to employment outside the home, education introduces another important source of differentiation between mothers and daughters. While most mothers in their forties and fifties are illiterate, most of the daughters have gone to school for 6–12 years. Not only does the school expose women to various discourses related to the body outside the domain of the family, but more importantly, literacy broadens the information available to young women. Books (religious and medical), magazines, and newspapers provide information related to maintaining, beautifying, and disciplining the body. The television set also introduces new ideas and products to clean, maintain, and beautify the body. Advertisements for shampoos, hair colors, and creams to whiten the skin stimulate desires for silkier, blonde hair and lighter face. Young women also have more access to places such as the beauty salon, which contribute to the shaping and regulation of the body.

At the same time, there are marked differences between female age groups in terms of displaying their beauty. While for young unmarried women beauty is central to their public identity and distinction, for older married women beauty should only be displayed in the domestic domain and they are not expected to show interest in their looks in front of others. Young single women are encouraged to care for their appearances and to beautify their bodies in ways that will receive acceptance and admiration from other people, especially men. The clothes they wear when they are out (libs khurug) are ironed, the face is carefully painted, and the hair is attentively styled. Money is saved to buy or rent clothes for special occasions such as weddings and religious feasts. Young women exchange clothes and put great effort into trying to match the colors of shoes and bags to their clothes. Parents, sisters, and friends encourage them to go to the hair salon, wear nice clothes, and dance in front of men and women at weddings, engagement celebrations, birthday parties, and other festive occasions.

Unlike young single women, married and older women are not expected to pay much attention to their looks in public. They are expected to beautify themselves only for their husbands. There seems to be, however, a strong decline in women's attention to their appearance after marriage and after the birth of their first child. One man, 'Ali, is in his mid-forties and runs a small shop in another low-income neighborhood but often visits his mother-in-law in Little Cairo. Although married for 18 years, he and his wife's sisters always point to the fact that his wife, unlike other married women, takes good care of herself. 'Ali described how women beautify themselves, fix their hair, and wear nice clothes and perfume before marriage. According to 'Ali, a man sees a young woman and he thinks she is "an angel that came down from the heavens." So he falls in love with her and works very hard to get engaged to her and then marry her. Then she gradually starts ignoring her looks and, as soon as she delivers her first child, she totally neglects herself and does not pay much attention to her husband's needs. The reason implied is that a woman feels 'secure' after having the first child and starts taking her husband for granted. 'Ali continues to say that the husband comes back home to find her in kitchen clothes, smelling of garlic, with messy hair and dirty clothes. This complaint is often voiced by men and young women (especially the husband's relatives) and is repeatedly discussed in television programs and soap operas. The wife is usually accused of neglecting herself and her husband. The discussions rarely bring up the competing time demands of housework, child-care, and time devoted to the husband. At the same time, critics do not link this tendency of married women with the general social attitude that discourages them from beautifying and displaying their bodies. One mother in her mid-forties living in Little Cairo explained that she feels embarrassed to wear makeup and nightgowns because her grownup sons do not approve. She shamefully remembers how her older son (in his early twenties) scolded her a few years ago for wearing lipstick and how she has stopped wearing it ever since, although she wore makeup before her children became adults.

Beauty and Identity

Several authors suggest that there is a strong link between self-identification and the maintenance and presentation of the body (Bourdieu 1984; Martin 1992; Gilman 1999). Erving Goffman presents an influential analysis of how the body mediates self-identity and social identity in the daily life. He argues that the self "is a performed character" and not "an organic thing that has a specific location . . . it is a dramatic effect arising diffusely from a scene that is presented, and the characteristic issue, the crucial concern, is whatever it will be credited or discredited" (Goffman 1959: 253). The body becomes a main vehicle in the performance of the self. "Body idioms" are "embodied expressive signs" that consist of "appearances and gestures" that communicate meanings about the self to others (Goffman 1963: 33–34). The mastery of these idioms, and other social skills linked to the management of the body, produce confidence and feelings of security. Timidity, embarrassment, and insecurity are the result of uneasiness towards the body and its collective representation, i.e., how it is seen by others, followed by attempts to correct the body and appropriate the social gaze in the formation of the legitimate body. These processes are best captured when looking at ideals of beauty and how they are negotiated and materialized. For many young women in Little Cairo, beauty is central to their self-identification. Beautiful women have distinction and social status.[4] They are praised by people and attract the gaze of both men and women. They are often the first to get married. A pretty wife usually has more power in dealing with her husband and with others. While married women quest for conception (to borrow the title of Marcia Inhorn's 1994 study on infertility in Egypt), unmarried young women quest for beauty. This is elaborated in the following pages, which focus the attention on the efforts of one young woman to acquire what is viewed as beautiful and desirable.

A Passion for Beauty: The Case of Jamila

When people in Little Cairo are asked to define beauty, they usually talk about the beauty of the soul (*halawit al-ruh*), good manners, and humor (*khafift al-damm*). Despite this emphasis on inner and substantive qualities, in daily life, physical appearances are always central to the description and evaluation of the beauty of others. For example, people in Little Cairo usually associate beauty with blond (*asfar*) hair, fair skin, and green eyes. The size and shape of the body are also part of the social construction of beauty. These views shape how young women perceive their bodies and how they try to rework certain parts of them to meet the expected social ideal.

As is the case in many other cultures (see, for example, Bordo 1995; Balsamo 1996), body beautification is related to disciplinary practices. Socially constructed ideals of beauty in Egypt are directly linked with female circumcision, removing facial hair, waxing legs and arms, using

---

4. In various cultures, beauty and attractiveness are associated with many positive qualities such as assertiveness, intelligence, fertility, and social value (Burke 1996). Beauty is also linked to employment decisions and in judging and predicting the behaviors of others. Unattractiveness, even in children, is usually linked to "aggressiveness," "antisocial behavior," and evil conduct (165).

makeup, and changing the color of the skin and the hair. Women in Little Cairo do not have access to plastic surgery or many other modern technologies used to modify the body (see, for example, Gilman 1999; Bordo 1995). Still, young women use various means to shape and beautify their bodies. The efforts of Jamila, an 18-year-old college student, exemplify how young women try to meet the expectations of others by using various strategies to beautify and reshape their bodies.

Like many of her peers, Jamila invests time and energy in beautifying and perfecting her body. She realizes the importance of what Bourdieu calls the "social gaze," which is "social power whose efficacy is always partly due to the fact that the receiver recognizes the categories of perception and appreciation it applies to him or her" (Bourdieu 1984: 207). The gaze of others is central to Jamila's self-identification and embodiment. She recognizes the values that people attach to various bodily forms and tries to meet social standards and emerging ideals of beauty. The reactions of others challenge or confirm her attempts at presenting a specific image of her body. Her hair, face, clothes, bags, and even shoes send messages about her financial abilities, taste, and distinction to the people in her community and at the college. Jamila's practices aim to attain certain ideals of beauty that are largely defined by people around her and by the flow of images and information through various media.

Jamila spends long hours thinking of ways to 'improve' and beautify her body. Similar to many other young women, Jamila pays special attention to certain parts of her body. The face and hair, for example, are main signifiers of beauty. The color and clarity of the skin, the color of the eyes, and the size of the mouth are especially important. The visibility of the face makes it central to people's judgments of others. One young woman expressed surprise at the fact that she cares so much for her own face. She goes to the doctor to get medication when there are pimples on her face and she buys expensive creams to whiten its skin. At the same time, she is reluctant to go to the doctor when she suffers from a vaginal infection that causes her great discomfort. Her face, she reasons, is seen by many and she feels a direct need to care for it. The emphasis on the face is also clearly manifested in marriage celebrations. Many brides stop wearing makeup and do not remove facial hair for weeks before their wedding day. This is done to make sure the bride 'glows' and looks more beautiful. The bride spends most of her wedding day in the beauty salon where her facial hair is removed and several masks are applied to whiten and clear the skin before applying full makeup.

Despite the fact that her facial features—large eyes, long eyelashes, high cheekbones, and a small mouth—are considered beautiful, Jamila focuses on changing and beautifying what is socially undesired. Her dark skin in particular is the source of her anxieties and discomfort. Skin color is one of the most important markers that people use to identify a person. Whiteness is highly appreciated. This is manifested among people in Little Cairo, who repeatedly say, "Even though she is white, she is not beautiful" and "Even though she is dark, she is beautiful." Beauty and whiteness are viewed as the norms while darkness and beauty are the exceptions. Jamila internalized the idea that white skin is beautiful and uses that to judge herself and others. She sees and hears various examples that exacerbate her insecurity about her relatively dark skin. Jamila's mother, for example, refused to allow her son to marry a young woman that he liked because her skin was dark (samra). "If my mother, who is herself dark and whose children are also dark, does this, how about other mothers whose children are whiter? Do you think they would want to chose someone like me?" Light skin is especially valued when it comes to women. Men are rarely judged by the color of their skin.

To be able to understand this preference for lighter skin, one needs to look at the history of race and the politics of color in Egypt.[5] It brings to the foreground issues related to class inequalities, the relationship between people from upper and lower Egypt, and conflicts between the Orient and the Occident. While documenting the history of this preference is beyond the scope of this paper, what interests me here is how this strong preference is central to the definition of beauty and the efforts of young women to beautify their skin. This desire structures Jamila's efforts and beauty-oriented practices. She uses different creams and masks (advertised on television, recommended by friends, physicians, pharmacists, hairdressers, and brought by her brother from the Gulf) to whiten her skin and remove blemishes and pimples. One cream she used was advertised on TV. The advertisement shows two young women who meet in a restaurant. They both look very beautiful with clear skin. One of them praises the other for looking even more beautiful than the last time she saw her. Teasingly, she asks "Does marriage make a woman so

5. This preference is common in different communities such as Sudan (Boddy 1997), Zimbabwe (Burke 1996), and the African-American community in the United States (Peiss 1998).

beautiful?" The other woman explains that she used Fair & Lovely cream for two weeks to whiten and clear her skin before her wedding. The first woman says that she will also used the same cream before her marriage. The advertisement makes a strong linkage between marriage (highly desirable among young women in Little Cairo) and light, clear skin. A beautiful bride is the one with clear skin and the women who are getting married are the ones with white skin. This linkage is important for Jamila. Most of her friends are either married or engaged. She feels that her delayed engagement is linked to her unattractive color. The advertisement increases her desire for a whiter skin and a chance for a match. She began using the cream. Jamila explains that at first it worked and her skin became lighter but it lost its effectiveness after a while. She continues to try other ways to achieve the white skin she desires.

Jamila noticed that one of their neighbors managed to whiten her skin and, according to Jamila, the neighbor became more beautiful. When asked, the neighbor said that she got a lotion from a female doctor who works at a clinic that is part of a local mosque. Jamila and her friends tried to get the prescription from the neighbor but she refused (because the neighbor is mean, according to Jamila) and told them to visit the doctor. Jamila visited the same doctor and got a prescription, which included a combination of products that were mixed in a local pharmacy. She used more than half her budget to buy the mixture needed to whiten her skin, but did not have enough money to buy the recommended sun block. Even though the doctor recommended that Jamila use the mixture only to whiten the skin of her neck, Jamila also applies it on her face. She was hopeful that this mixture would be more effective than the other creams but that is yet to be seen.

The market for beauty products also includes pharmacists and hairdressers, who actively market various kinds of oils and mixtures to whiten the skin. The hairdresser recommended a mask that Jamila, her sister, sister-in-law, and other friends used to remove pimples, dark spots, and to whiten the skin. I was with Jamila one day when a pharmacist assured her that he got a new cream from England that will be very effective in whitening her skin. He emphasized that he obtained a limited quantity of the cream for his wife and had only a few extra tubes left. Jamila bought a tube hoping that this imported cream would work better than locally produced products.

These various creams peel Jamila's skin. In several cases, her cheeks became red, most likely a sign of skin irritation. People around her saw these cheeks as a sign of beauty that elicited both compliments and reprimands. In high school, she was asked by the teachers to wash her face to make sure that she was not using makeup. I was with her when a religious jeweler scolded her because he claimed that it was forbidden (*haram*) for her to color her cheeks. The redness of her cheeks was also complimented by her friends and colleagues at school, who tried to learn the secret of her rosy cheeks. Such compliments motivate Jamila to continue her search for a better cream with long-lasting effects.

Acquiring a light skin is part of Jamila's attempts to 'pass.' According to Sander Gilman, passing indicates a desire to be visible (i.e., belong to a desirable cohort) and invisible (i.e., not clearly differentiated from this desirable group). She is trying to belong to what is viewed as more beautiful and desirable. In this endeavor, Jamila has other body parts to worry about. Her long, straight, soft hair is considered beautiful compared to curly or wavy hair. She carefully washes her hair with shampoo and soaks it with oil either bought from a local store or brought by one of her brothers from the Gulf. But her dark hair color is not considered beautiful so she uses different dyes to make it blond. She tried a color that she saw on television, which was for her relatively expensive (around £E 6 out of her £E 10 weekly allowance). She decided to pay its high price because it did not contain ammonia and peroxide, which dry the hair. She was disappointed when the hair color remained too dark. So she bought ammonia and a dye from a nearby shop for £E 0.50. This color did not last so she had to dye her hair a third time two days later to get the color that she wanted.

Jamila does not like the fact that she is taller than all her sisters, friends, and some of her brothers. She feels that a woman should be delicate (*ra'i'a*) and not tall like men. She tries to downplay her height by increasing her weight. One of her friends introduced her to a medicine that is available in a local pharmacy. This drug, according to her description, retains the water in the body and makes the face look round and the body full. She also took another medicine to stimulate her appetite and, according to her sister, Jamila started eating without stopping. When comparing her pictures before and after taking the medicine, the difference was tremendous. Her face looked rounder in one of the pictures and less so in other pictures. She was sad while looking at her pictures. "Look how beautiful my face was? It was also much whiter when it was full and round (*midawwar*)." Several other young women were also using the drug. She pointed to one of them, Safia, who was skinny but after taking the drug, her cheeks became full *(malyana)*. Safia, according to Jamila, became so beautiful that she immediately got engaged. She had to stop taking the medicine before getting married because she heard rumors that it may cause infertility. Jamila herself believes that the drug causes infertility and encourages her friends to stop using it a few months before marrying. She experienced irregularities with her period. The flow became less, the color of the blood darkened, and her usual cramps stopped. It is widely believed (and often supported by local physicians) that menstrual cramps signal that the ovaries are active. Hence, young women usually refuse to take medication to stop the pain. For Jamila and many other women, fertility takes clear priority over beauty.

Many of the activities that Jamila and her friends engage in are done without the knowledge of their mothers. Books, magazines, and prescriptions for a drug or a new lotion are circulated among young women away from the gaze of others. Jamila did not tell her mother that she was taking a medicine that retained water in her body. She and her older sister thought that their mother would be very upset if she heard about the drug, which caused Jamila's subsequent sickness. After three months of taking the drug, Jamila's kidneys started causing her pain while the rest of her body swelled so much that she was not able to bend her hands or to do her daily chores. According to Jamila, the doctor recognized her problem immediately. He scolded her and said that this problem is common among women in Little Cairo. He explained to her the risks associated with taking the drug and gave her medication that is used to treat some serious kidney diseases. She felt better after a while but did not feel any desire to eat. So, the physician gave her another medicine to stimulate her appetite. She is gaining weight every day and is surprised when people tell her that she is becoming fat *(takhina)*. She asks me and others whether she is really fat or just full *(malyana)*, two different conditions, the second of which is the desired one.

Is Plumpness Beautiful? Competing Constructions

While for many mothers, the plump body signals beauty and status (see Ghannam 1997), the situation is more complicated for many of their daughters. Older women link plumpness with beauty ·and sexual desirability. Men, women often believe, prefer plump figures. Preference for the plump body, however, is not as strong as it was a generation ago. Young educated men, especially those who have worked abroad and have had the chance to interact with people outside their neighborhood, tend to see beauty in slender figures. The image of the slim body is competing with (though still far from displacing) the ideal of the plump body when selecting a wife. Older men are also questioning the beauty of the plump body. While watching TV with me, his wife, and one of his wife's friends, a man in his late fifties who works as a mechanic in Little Cairo commented on the fact that Latifa, a popular Tunisian singer, has gained weight by declaring that fat women are 'worthless.' The comment came as a criticism of his wife and her friend since both of them have gained weight over the years. His wife, who often prides herself on her plump body, was shocked by his statement. She tried to hide her disappointment by jokingly accusing him of desiring a slimmer woman. Her female friend interjected by declaring that neither her husband nor her friend's husband was slender, and therefore they should not criticize their wives. Rather than agreeing with her, the wife announced that men's 'fatness' was good while women's 'fatness' was bad. This encounter summarizes how criticism of one's weight is often directed at women and not at men. New markers are emerging to reinforce the gendered character of the body. While, as clear in the introduction to this chapter, female newscasters are criticized for gaining weight and are 'encouraged' to stay slim, male newscasters are not forced to lose weight. Similarly, men in Little Cairo are not criticized for their fat bellies. Only fat on the female body is increasingly seen as undesirable.

Young women in Little Cairo are under contradictory pressures to present their bodies and shape them in ways that are considered socially appropriate, healthy, and beautiful. Their mothers argue that they need a certain amount of fat to look beautiful while there are many other images that emphasize the slender figure. Jamila and many other young women try to work these images and differences in various ways. The issue for many of them is not simply to lose or gain weight. Rather, it is gaining and losing weight in the right places. Young women try different ways to lose weight. Some use acupuncture, other take drugs to suppress their appetite or go on diets. Some shift from dark to light soft drinks (i.e., from Coca-Cola to Seven Up). Some go to clinics and gyms. Through these methods, young women are trying to combine old and new ideals of the plump and slender body. A young woman who gains too much weight and has a tummy (kirsh) and buttocks (hansh) is seen as a married woman (madame) who has given birth. This is not desirable. So, young women face the challenge of gaining weight and losing weight in the right places. The rounded face is very much desired by many young women. Several young women described how happy they feel when their faces become rounder without weight gain around their tummies and buttocks. They expressed distress and unhappiness when their faces get thinner. Young women try to achieve the praised figure of *malfufa* (from the word *laff*, which means, among other things, to make rounded) and *mit'assimma* (from the verb *qassam*, which means to divide, indicating clear curves and contours). These two words refer to the rounded body and its plumpness in the right places, which include a big bust, slim belly and behind, and a clearly defined waistline. The preference for the body that is *malfuf* or *mit'assim* is linked with wearing 'modern' cloths. While the *gallabiya*, a loose full-length garb, does not reveal the contours of the body, the skirt and the blouse reveal various details of the figure. These two styles of clothes also mark differences between older and younger women. The former tend to wear *gallabiya*s most of the time while the latter tend to wear skirts and pants.

Differences between mothers and daughters signal the presence of different ideals for the construction of feminine identity. Unlike her daughter, Jamila's mother, a widow in her mid-fifties, pays attention to her body primarily because of medical and religious reasons. She suffers from high blood pressure and hemorrhoids. In addition to regular visits to local clinics and observation of food and medicine intakes, Umm Jamila pays a great deal of attention to her dress code to match her religious devotion. Her interest in bodily hygiene is often given religious meanings. Bathing, washing, and dressing her body are linked to prayer and going to the mosque. Socially, she is not expected to pay attention to her appearance. More than the beauty of her face, it is her role as a mother and her religious piety that shape her identity. For Jamila, due to age, education, aspirations, and marital status, her looks play a central role in the construction of her gendered identity.

Young women are not only struggling with the more old-fashioned preferences of their mothers but they also have to negotiate various religious discourses in the formation of their bodies. There are religious debates about various aspects of the female body that range from shaping the eyebrows and using makeup to abortion and family planning. For Jamila and many of her friends, religion is one powerful and competing discourse among many that shape their bodies. Jamila is very critical of her unmarried, 24-year-old sister, Laila, who is not making similar efforts to whiten her skin and beautify her face and hair. "Look at the area under her eyes. It is so dark. She does not try to take care of herself." Laila uses makeup to beautify her face and she pays a great deal of attention to her clothes. She carefully shapes her eyebrows and removes hair from her face, legs, and arms. She covers her curly hair with colorful head covers and uses makeup to whiten her face skin. Laila, who tried some masks and creams but quickly was frustrated by their ineffectiveness, gives religious meanings to her unwillingness to do what Jamila does. She says "Jamila is not content with what God gave her. She feels that she needs to become more beautiful. But I feel that she is trying to change God's creation, something that I disagree with." Jamila, however, does not see any contradiction between her passion for beauty and any religious values. She emphasizes that one day she will cover her hair but she does not see that as an urgent priority.

Emerging Discourses and Gendered Bodies

This paper aimed to elaborate on four points: First, class, as Pierre Bourdieu argues, plays a central role in shaping bodily preferences and ideals of beauty. However, there is much more flexibility and room for improvisation in this process than indicated in my analysis. Second, although often marginalized in Bourdieu's model, gender is a very important dimension that intersects with class in powerful ways to shape perceptions of the body. Third, unlike what is suggested by Carol Delaney, women within the same socioeconomic background may internalize multiple constructions of the body. Fourth, the globalization of economy and culture is introducing new desires and possibilities for shaping the body. Jamila, Farida El-Zommor, and Samia Alluba are all struggling with different views about their bodies and how they should be presented. Jamila was trying to change her body into one that is socially valued and desired. She wanted to match several ideals of beauty and has been trying to perfect her body to meet the expectations of the people around her. She tried to whiten her face and neck to meet the general preference for white skin. She aimed to change the color of her hair from dark to blond while retaining its preferred straightness. She resented the fact that she was taller than all her friends, viewing tallness as a male quality. She tried to compensate for that by gaining weight. She wanted to become more feminine by keeping her long hair and by wearing skirts and dresses instead of pants. Jamila depends on the gaze of others and notices their reactions to her efforts. These reactions confirm or challenge the changes she introduced to her body. Praise for her rosy cheeks encourages her to work harder to find creams that promise to whiten her skin. Being referred to by others (such as her brother-in-law) as getting fat while being praised by her mother for her full body puts contradictory demands on Jamila. She changes her strategies depending on the reaction of her friends and relatives. She continuously reconsiders her efforts based on the reactions of others.

Jamila's views of her body are closely linked with the flow of information that stimulates different desires and a market of beauty products that promises to materialize these desires. At one level, the female body is under the control of the family and the community, especially when it comes to issues related to sexuality and reproduction (Ghannam 1997). The above discussion, however, shows how this control is not total. Education and the circulation of information are providing young women with spaces to shape their bodies in ways that are not controlled by their families. The efforts of Jamila and her friends are informed by socially constructed ideals of beauty and by emerging views and products. There is a flourishing market for products that young women like Jamila use to beautify their bodies. Jamila's desire for a socially perfect body continues to take her to doctors, hairdressers, and pharmacists. Her efforts are not materialized in long-term achievements. Her skin is whitened for a short time after using a mask or a cream but quickly returns to its darker shade. Her efforts do not overcome the constraints imposed by her body and the restrictions of her budget. But she tries again and again.

Bibliography

Balsamo, Anne, 1996, *Technologies of the Gendered Body: Reading Cyborg Women*. Durham: Duke University Press.

Boddy, Janice, 1997, "The Womb as Oasis: The Symbolic Context of Pharaonic Circumcision in Rural Northern Sudan," *The Gender/Sexuality Reader*, Roger Lancaster and Micaela di Leonardo, eds., 309–324. London: Routledge.

Bordo, Susan, 1995, *Unbearable Weight: Feminism, Western Culture, and the Body*. Berkeley: University of California Press.

Bourdieu, Pierre, 1977, *Outline of a Theory of Practice*. Cambridge: Cambridge University Press.

———, 1984, *Distinction: A Social Critique of the Judgement of Taste*. London: Routledge.

———, 1990, *The Logic of Practice*. Stanford: Stanford University Press.

Burke, Timothy, 1996, *Lifebuoy Men, Lux Women: Commodification, Consumption, and Cleanliness in Modern Zimbabwe*. Durham: Duke University Press.

de Certeau, Michel, 1988, *The Practice of Everyday Life*. Berkeley: University of California Press.

Delaney, Carol, 1991, *The Seed and the Soil: Gender and Cosmology in Turkish Village Society*. Berkeley: University of California Press.

Featherstone, Mike, Mike Hepworth, and Bryan Turner, 1991, The Body: Social Process and Cultural Theory. London: Sage Publications.

Foucault, Michel, 1979, *Discipline and Punish: The Birth of the Prison*. New York: Vintage Books.

———, 1980, *The History of Sexuality*. New York: Vintage Books.

———, 1990, *The Use of Pleasure*. New York: Vintage Books.

Frank, Arthur W., 1991, "For a Sociology of the Body: An Analytical Review," *The Body, Social Process and Cultural Theory*, Mike Featherstone, Mike Hepworth, and Brayn S. Turner, eds., 36–102. London: Sage Publications.

Ghannam, Farha, 1997, "Fertile, Plump, and Strong: The Social Construction of the Female Body in Low-income Cairo." Monograph. Cairo: The Reproductive Health Working Group, the Population Council.

Gilman, Sander, 1999, *Making the Body Beautiful: A Cultural History of Aesthetic Surgery*. Princeton: Princeton University Press.

———, 1998, *Making the Body Beautiful: A Cultural History of Aesthetic Surgery*. Princeton: Princeton University Press.

Goffman, Erving, 1959, *The Presentation of the Self in Everyday Life*. New York: Double Day Archer Books.

———, 1963, *Behavior in Public Places: Notes on the Social Organization of Gatherings*. London: The Free Press of Glencoe.

Good, Byron J., 1994, *Medicine, Rationality, and Experience*. Cambridge: Cambridge University Press.

Grosz, Elizabeth, 1994, *Volatile Bodies: Toward a Corporeal Feminism*. Indianapolis: Indiana University Press.

Harker, Richard, Cheleen Maher, and Chris Wilkes, eds., 1990, *An Introduction to the Work of Pierre Bourdieu*. London: Macmillan Press.

Inhorn, Marcia Claire, 1994, *Quest for Conception: Gender, Infertility, and Egyptian Medical Traditions*. Philadelphia: University of Pennsylvania.

———, 1996, *Infertility and Patriarchy: The Cultural Politics of Gender and Family in Egypt*. Philadelphia: University of Pennsylvania.

Martin, Emily, 1992, *The Woman in the Body: A Cultural Analysis of Reproduction*. Boston: Beacon.

Peiss, Kathy, 1998, "Women Who Painted," "Promoting Made-up Women," and "Identity and the Market," *Hope in a Jar: The Making of America's Beauty Culture*, 37–60, 134–164, 238–269. New York: Metropolitan Books.

Shilling, Chris, 1993, *The Body and Social Theory*. London: Sage Publications.

Synnott, Anthony, 1992, "Tomb, Temple, Machine, and Self: The Social Construction of the Body," *British Journal of Sociology*, 43 (1): 79–110.

———, 1993, *The Body Social: Symbolism, Self and Society*. London: Routledge.

Turner, Bryan S., 1984, *The Body and Society, Explorations in Social Theory*. Oxford: Basil Blackwell.

———, 1991, "Review Article: Missing Bodies: Towards a Sociology of Embodiment," *Sociology of Health & Illness*, 13 (2): 265–272.

———, 1991a, "Recent Developments in the Theory of the Body," *The Body, Social Process, and Cultural Theory*, Mike Featherstone, Mike Hepworth, and Brayn S. Turner, eds., 1–35. London: Sage Publications.

———, 1992, *Regulating Bodies: Essays in Medical Anthropology*. New York: Routledge.

Fi nas wi fi nas

Class Culture and Illness Practice in Egypt

MONTASSER M. KAMAL

Human activity can never be considered outside of the framework of social relations and their history, which provide the logic of social activity—its rhyme and reason. The meaning of activity cannot, therefore, be considered purely in terms of symbolically constructed meaning, nor with reference only to activity we cannot interpret the actions or the motives of individuals simply by seeking out the meaning that has inspired their activity. Rather, we must set activity and the individual accounts given of actions and motives in the context of their social logic: that is of social relations and social activity as a whole (Burkitt 1991: 194).

Logic, Perception, and Practice

It is often said that in the Middle East group affiliation is considered superior to an individual-centered existence. This formulation has been central to discussions of Egyptian and Arab culture over the past several decades. The claim for importance of group affiliation comes from empirical observation and from the way 'natives' speak of themselves. This representation is found in studies of history, sociology, anthropology, political science, and other social sciences (see Patai 1973; Rugh 1984; Early 1993; Tucker 1993; Wikan 1996).

One might question the extent to which this limited formulation adequately represents or ever represented the nuances of affiliation in contemporary Egyptian culture. An equally important question, which is posed in this chapter, is to ask: what does this formulation mask? One answer might be to cite an Egyptian saying: *Fi nas wi fi nas*, which translates as "There are people and then there are (other) people." Among the most familiar interpretations of this saying is that people are not equal: there are differences based on social standing, economic status, or class. This view proposes that the

> oriental formation is a hierarchical one. There are exploited
> strata and exploiting strata . . . not to mention the role of the
> state . . . which practices oppression under the name of society,
> or in other terms for the benefit of the dominating stratum
> (Siam 1995: 76–77, author's translation).

A narrow representation of social relations is further complicated. Group affiliation is often reduced—by Egyptian and foreign authors, and also social scientists—to kinship. Kinship is central to individual and social identification, but reductionism masks understanding other forms of group affiliation. Consequently, people's everyday life practices are not seen as a product of a more dynamic interaction of personal, social, and ideological elements. Thus the study of social affiliation is masked by abstract—as well as familial—studies of social organization in Egypt and the Arab World (Gad 1994, 1995a, 1995b). These studies also usurp the study of intra-class relations for a more conventional study of inter-class differences. Subsequently, consciousness of individuals as regards their social, cultural, and national identity and life strategies are rarely represented.

This chapter will show how people's affiliation in Egypt must be situated within the personal as well as the social and ideological organization of the entire society as a prerequisite for studying their ways of dealing with compromised health. For this purpose, I will rely somewhat on Pierre Bourdieu's concepts of class habitus and capital. These points will be illustrated in this chapter based on data from a 1995–1996 fieldwork in the Cairo neighborhood of Sayyida Zaynab.[1]

---

1. This study benefited from the financial support of an MEAward #335 granted by the Population Council, West Asia and North Africa, for the period of 1995–1996. This research would not have been possible without the facilitation provided by the Near East Foundation/Center for Development Services, Cairo. A grant from the Ford Foundation has made writing the research results possible. The views presented here are entirely mine.

Social Location and Practice

Reflecting on the work of Bourdieu, it has been noted that the 'logic of practice' of everyday life, is completely internalized, without being questioned, but practice "is not without its purpose or practical intent" (Williams 1995: 582). People are immersed in a habitus, which structures and forms their experiential being in the world (Bourdieu 1984, 1990). Thus habitus provides individuals with class-dependent 'naturalized' ways of classifying the social world and their location within it (Williams 1995: 585–6; Postone et al. 1993: 4).

The concept of class habitus will be employed here to demonstrate that not only relations of kinship but also an individual's class and social location inculcate a person with naturalized modes of practice that are manifested in both instrumental and emotional coping with illness. Class habitus refers to a mix of social dispositions that are instilled in the person. These dispositions are based on social stratifications that are further reproduced through social actions and interaction, which are in themselves delimited, based on the person's class habitus. In Egyptian society, the saying *fi nas wi fi nas* is an indigenous way of portraying people's perceptions— and actions—that is intimately linked to the concept of class habitus.

The ethnographic data presented here, however, will show a departure from Bourdieu's view that a person's

> actions and works are the product of a modus operandi of which he is not the producer and has no conscious mastery. . . . The scheme of thought and expression he has acquired are the basis for this intentionless invention of regulated improvisation (Bourdieu 1977: 79).

In the Egyptian context, illness practice—a term that will become clearer below—allows us to observe that a person's dispositions can also be purposefully and consciously reproduced. In other words, that being an Egyptian engaged in social—or illness—practice is not only a matter of tacit knowledge. As Moore points out, "social systems consist of social practices situated in space–time and produced and reproduced through the actions of knowledgeable social actors" (Moore 1996: ix).

For Bourdieu, a class habitus is directly linked to capital of which there are at least two categories: material and immaterial (Calhoun 1993). Material capital refers to the financial capital available for the purchase of commodities and products, and is based on the rules of the marketplace.

Immaterial capital includes mainly cultural capital (e.g., education), social capital (e.g., social relations and networks), but also symbolic capital (e.g., "reputation for competence and an image of respectability and honorability" [Bourdieu 1984: 291]).[2] Of the immaterial capital, the concepts of social and cultural capital have been more frequently employed.

During this research, I observed how some individuals from a certain social group decide that others in it have more or less of a given amount of capital. Alternatively, they may conclude that certain individuals should not be included in their level/standard or social category, and that consequently their life and illness practices should not cross paths. According to Bourdieu, this could be attributed to a different composition of capital within class habitus, which might consist of a combination of economic, social, and cultural capital. What is proposed here, however, is that these differences, and consequent illness practice are best understood as locally produced and historically constituted, creating a particular 'culture' for each group that can be termed a 'subculture.' What Bourdieu calls "secondary properties" can best be termed, then, as 'subcultural properties' of social groups.[3]

Hence it is possible to postulate a definition—that will be refined at the end of this chapter—of illness practice as "the outward expression of culturally constructed perceptions of wellness and illness that are structurally grounded. It entails both perception and practice or cognition and action that are, at once, consciously and unconsciously produced by and reproduce the objective and subjective heterogeneity in society." Illness practice like other social practice, sometimes confirms, sometimes challenges, and sometimes accommodates the social world. But, in all cases, as will be shown below, it reveals the internalized perceptions of social order. My attempt is close to the view that:

---

2. The term "physical capital" has also been referred to by Bourdieu (Williams 1995: 587). The concept refers to the body as a resource to be employed to meet different ends, including recreation.

3. Despite this proposed refinement, a gap remains in Bourdieu's work. His work stops short of analysis of gender differences in class habitus and in terms of availability and/or control over capital. While this limits the possibility of invoking generalizations based on his approach, it does not affect its validity in understanding some of the shared structural parameters of everyday life.

most passing on and subsequent affirmation of culture take place in the course of interested actions in which people pursue a variety of ends, both conscious and unconscious (Calhoun 1993: 78).

Subcultures and Social Stratification

In Egypt, illness practice works through a subculture developed within a given class habitus, which is mediated through social networks controlling the societal distribution of resources. Subculture is a form of social relations that exists in a matrix of specific cultural norms and social organization, which get expressed in language, non-verbal expressions, customs, aesthetics, and relational values employed to (re)create a particular form of social organization. Attempts to capture this refinement in the context of Egypt have had limitations.

Janet Abu-Lughod proposes the existence of three sub-cities or sub-areas in Cairo, which correspond to the three urban worlds of the rural, the traditional urban, and the modern urban. She points out that the "style of life" in each of these sub-cities is distinguishable on the basis of socioeconomic variables and patterns of social relationships (Abu-Lughod 1971). I would like to propose that what she is coining as a "style of life" is indeed better termed a subculture. The residents of the sub-cities indeed have a consciously drawn line of demarcation between them and the 'other.' Socioeconomic variations in the urban experience more than create particular living conditions, they create the moral and material world of social differentiation (see Early 1993; Wikan 1996) that produce the specificity of a subculture.

El Missiri Nadim proposes that the residents of the *hara* (an alley or narrow street in a traditional neighborhood) have their own subculture because they "share certain historical, ecological, and sociocultural experiences which point to an identifiable style of life" (El Missiri Nadim 1975: 200). Their way of life is indeed a "subculture within the larger cultural system of Cairo and Egypt" (201). Hence, a concept of subculture is potentially useful more than that of a "style of life" to explain heterogeneity in social positions and dispositions. The concept gives weight to pluralistic social interaction and value systems as means of linking perception with practice. In this situation, perceptions of 'self' and 'other' are very much part of the work of culture to produce personal and group identity (see Obeyesekere 1990). A subculture is a form of cultural identity that is based on perceptions operative in a particular dominant culture. In agreement with Homi Bhabha, it is important to note that the creation of a cultural identity is not free from relationships of class, power, and authority, and indeed ambivalence (Bhabha 1990a; 1990b).

In other words, a study of social structure without the study of perceptions and practice within it leads to misrepresentation of cultural complexity. Understanding illness practice then requires a better understanding of the link between class habitus and culture. In the case of Egypt, social classes have always evolved as social structures of differentiated cultural values and informed by an ethos of national progress and modernity. Regrettably in Egypt, the already scarce studies of social interaction in health and illness take place in a social class vacuum.

Soheir A. Morsy quotes a villager as saying: "I wish we could live like the city. I wish we could live there [with] all the electricity and water. . . . People in the city have more money, they buy meat at least once a week, not like us. I wish I was born in the city; I would have gone to school and learned to read and write" (Morsy 1993: 211). This villager, in addition to his or her individual aspirations, shares a commonly held aspiration more fundamental than a change in residence or lifestyle—a structural change into another class and subsequently a class habitus. These aspirations are part of "social, political, and spiritual processes of life" which are determined by modes of production or "social existence" (Marx and Engels 1971: 16). Social and ideological concepts are inculcated in people and are evident in their aspirations, even if not expressed in their discursive exchange: "For the peasants . . . although the language of class is not part of their vocabulary, and neither is the rhetoric of [gender] equality . . . the consequences of their status as peasants are anything but understated" (Morsy 1993: 192).

Historically, the state in Egypt has been the creator of social classes, through transformation of relationships of production and taxation, control of institutions of social welfare and well-being, and by acting as the main benefactor/protector of social order and resources (Marsot 1984; Kuhnke 1990; Gad 1995a, 1995b).[4] Furthermore,

---

4. The Egyptian bourgeoisie has traditionally been allied with the west and their assets were equally divided between the agricultural and industrial spheres (Zaalouk 1989: 23). Neither during the nineteenth-century economic and legal reforms, nor during the inter-war and post-World War II periods did the Egyptian bourgeoisie emerge as a result of a class struggle similar to that of the west (Tignor 1982).

while changes in modes of production have historically influenced class stratification in Egypt, socionaturalization of classes was accomplished through the integration of class structure into individual perceptions and social practices.

The second half of the twentieth century witnessed the assault on conventional class structure in Egypt under Gamal Abd al-Nasser's socialist regime and Anwar Sadat's Open Door economic policies and economic liberalization (Ajami 1982; Dessouki 1982; Zaalouk 1989; Imam 1991; Morsy 1993; Gad 1994, 1995b; Noweer 1994). In all stages, economic means were closely linked to perceptions and actions that further reveal the class habitus of individuals and groups in society, with very limited mobility: "[F]rom the late 1960s on, the class struc-ture appears to have been hardening again . . . upward mobility has increasingly become "confined" to children of the middle and upper strata. For younger members of the lowers rungs, such opportunities are to be found outside the Egyptian system" (Ibrahim 1982: 431).

Additionally, belonging to one class and being ascribed another by virtue of affiliation, or being ascribed a certain class by virtue of being a woman or wife (Fergani 1994), does not make class categorization in Egypt a neat pursuit.[5] The expression of a social class, born through means of production, is most evident in the domain of practice. Probably one of the most informing arenas of the study of class and culture in Egypt is that of dealing with compromised health.

Distinction in Illness Practice

The relationship between capitalism and ill health is not to "be attrib-uted simply to capitalism in any crude sense" (Doyal 1979: 27, 1995). It has already been established that social class determines the environmental conditions in which people live and their access to serv-ices in healthcare, including referrals and consultations (Morgan et al. 1985: 219–220; Blane 1982). Hence, inequalities in health exist as a

---

5. Most studies on the subject have suffered from mimicking lines of inquiry formulated to understand the nineteenth-century capitalist transition in Europe, which deflects from the cultural specificity in Arab society (Gad 1994). Dependency on western theories and models, and the inability to reach a con-sensus on which means of production predominated in the modern history of Egypt (Gad 1994) make a dynamic study of class, culture, and illness practice a formidable task.of a class struggle similar to that of the west (Tignor 1982).

"product of the differences in their life situations and this reflects the priorities and nature of the wider socioeconomic system" (233).[6]

Equally, in more subdued ways, managing illness is a result of a fundamentally class-linked set of perceptions and practices. For instance, let us take the doctor-patient relationship as an element of illness practice. Lisbeth Sachs (1989) proposes that negotiation of an outcome in a medical encounter is based on a negotiation of differing cultural and medical traditions, and culturally valued expectations. Wayne Katon and Arthur Kleinman propose that negotiation becomes an "integral part of the primary care physician's work, a core clinical task" (Katon and Kleinman 1981: 276). Rose Wiles and Joan Higgins' proposed perceptions of doctor-patient encounters have changed from paternalism to more of a "mutuality and consumerism." (Wiles and Higgins 1996)

It is hard to imagine that, for example, in Sri Lanka peasants do not go to the doctor carrying their social class with them in their consciousness, their practice, and their expectations (see Singer 1987). Equally hard to grasp is that in England, "consumerism and mutuality" between doctors and patients are separate from a more generalized class texture of society. According to Bourdieu: "The individuals grouped in a class that is constructed in a particular respect . . . always bring with them, in addition to their pertinent properties by which they are classified, secondary properties which are thus smuggled into the explanatory model" (Bourdieu 1984: 102).

In these cases, one is left with the false impression that an outcome of illness practice may actually improve through technical knowledge and skills (see Katon and Kleinman 1981).[7] Understanding illness practice then must also be situated within a framework of sociocultural beliefs that must be further integrated within a more profound

---

6. The relationship between class, disease, and illness is explored more in sociology than in anthropology (e.g., Doyal 1979; Blane 1982; Eyer 1984; Morgan et al. 1985).

7. This false impression produces a controversial view that giving more control to patients is separable from necessary attempts to address the deeper foundation of economic and ideological stratification in society (Singer 1987). Additionally, this implies that sensitization or even incorporation of a sociopolitical perspective in medical training and encounters as proposed by Mary-Jo Delvecchio Good and Byron J. Good (1982) is sufficient.

view that "many of the conditions the patients bring to medical settings have their origins in the way in which society is organized—in socially arranged work and leisure activities and their distribution among persons of different 'races,' genders, social classes, and religious and cultural backgrounds" (Hahn 1995: 171).

It remains to be answered how social class influences the cultural basis of illness practice. As we shall see, illness practice happens in many cases despite the logic of social class affiliation and not always in accordance with it. The relation between social class and illness practice is thus not a rational, linear one. It is a problematic one because although it is informed by social class stratification, it is predicated also on intra-class relations. To belong to one class does not mean sharing the same subculture.

It will take more than this study to refine the representation of the inter-linkages between perceptions and practices within a sociocultural and structural framework class. However, this chapter will present narratives of people whose self-representation reveals more on class culture in illness practice than usually captures attention.

Illness Narratives

Ayman's 'Us'

Ayman is a 26-year-old university graduate. Both his parents are teachers, one in a secondary school and the other in a preparatory school. His parents moved to Cairo from Ismailia, 100 kilometers east of Cairo along the Suez Canal, after the 1967 war and before Ayman was born. His father owns a ten-feddans farm turned into a rented-out fruit orchard in Ismailia. Ayman finished his studies at the faculty of commerce and is currently enrolled in the military to complete his obligatory service. He is enrolled as an 'officer,' which means he will have to stay in active service for three years, after which he will be on reserve for a few more years. At the time, he was completing his last year of military service. As a conscript, his pay is nominal.

Ayman tells the story of how six months ago he came back home from the Red Sea, where he is stationed, with the following complaint:

> I was not able to lift my right arm as before. I found it very
> difficult to carry anything even if it is not heavy, even if for one
> minute. . . . I had numbness in most of my arm. It was worse just
> after I woke up and before I went to sleep at night. . . . For two or

three weeks I thought perhaps I had squeezed my arm under my body in my sleep, or I had struck my arm against something, or even carried something too heavy as we often do in the military . . . but after a few weeks, I realized that the numbness was not going away. . . . The numbness started to go higher in my arm that it was almost up to the middle of my arm [the middle of his biceps], but after a while it neither increased nor decreased.

Ayman adds that he was then beset with numbness in the back of his neck, recalling:

I was so scared, I thought maybe this numbness was going to spread all over my body. . . . I was scared that it would spread to other parts of my body. . . . I stayed up all night waiting for it to go away. . . . I only fell asleep when I was exhausted . . . then I would wake up at dawn to find it was still there. . . . It did not go away. . . . It was 'clutching' in my neck like a big, strong fist.

Existential and perceptual, Ayman's experience is not restricted to his body sensation. The perceptual aspects are culturally constructed through social interaction within a particular social organization. Ayman's numbness is indeed as much a cultural experience as a physical one. To understand this, we need to listen more to what he has to say.

After the first few days of the incidence of the numbness in my right hand I told one of my friends with me in the military camp. . . . I only met him [for the first time] in the camp. We often shared duties and shifts. This made it easier on both of us. . . . It always helps to have someone you like, someone who understands who you are and what you want. . . . I told him about my hand. He told me it is probably nothing: "It will go away. Maybe it is [because of] something heavy you carried without paying attention."

His friend Mahmoud is Ayman's age. He has a degree in law. He is the son of a mid-level government manager. His mother is a housewife. He and his two school-age sisters live with their parents. Ayman recounted that Mahmoud would regularly ask about his arm. He even told him to do a certain exercise that would make him feel better. Ayman added:

I did not want to tell anyone else. Sometimes it was so numb that I thought I had lost all sensation in my arm, but I still did not want to tell anyone. . . . You know, the other guys in the camp are not really friends, they will think that I am faking it. . . . Also, many of them come from a poor bi'ah (environment), not even from Cairo. If I tell anyone, the news will spread and they will all make fun of me and talk behind me and in front of me about 'being like a girl.' I prefer not to share this problem with these people. I discussed it with Mahmoud, my friend, and decided that it is better to just go to a doctor next time during my vacation, which was coming a few days later.

On returning home, Ayman's father told him: "Why didn't you speak to your superior? He could have given you time off, or given you a permit to go the military doctor or hospital." This contrasted with his mother's perspective:

Military hospitals in the Red Sea are useless. I am sure they would have just given him aspirin and told him to go back to his camp. They probably have a ghalban (humble, poor) doctor. I will speak to your uncle (her brother). He has a neurologist's clinic one floor above his apartment. . . . I will ask him to book an appointment for us. . . . I know that you would have not gotten anything out of that Red Sea doctor.

Ayman's illness practice was practically charted out for him. As if all he had to do is feel something, express it, and leave its interpretation largely for others. His condition is located in his body, but the full extent of his experience is also situated elsewhere, in the bodies of others—kin and non-kin—around him, in their class habitus, and in Egypt's healthcare system.

Ayman is situated within a class habitus, which processes social and cultural signals and internalizes them into social roles, values, and practice. However, this homogeneity in the outlook of life masks a subculture of disharmony, as will become clearer later. His experience was located in his class habitus subculture. His physical discomfort and pain passed through culturally constructed class and other social filters which finally dictated how culturally salient his presentation of illness can be (Good 1994; Kleinman et al. 1994). Now let us see if the class dynamics of women's illness practice is different.

Amina's Burden

Amina is a 28-year-old graduate of the faculty of education. She has been married for four years. She has an 18-month-old daughter and a three-year-old son. She was pregnant at the time of the interview. Amina is the daughter of the general manager of the personnel department of one of the government ministries in Cairo. Her mother has not completed her educucation and has never worked outside the house. The parents own a four-story building (*bait*). The family has been living in this bait for more than forty years. The upper two floors are inhabited by two of the offspring; Amina lives on the third floor with her family, and her brother Salem on the top floor with his family. The ground floor is rented out to shops.

In the third month of her pregnancy Amina experienced some discomfort:

> Last Ramadan I was sitting after the kids went to sleep to watch television and waiting for Gamal [her husband] to come home. I was so tired so I did not go down to [visit] my parents and also the kids were already asleep. . . . I felt like I was having a discharge. I got up and went to the bathroom. . . . I checked myself. . . . I found some blood, I got worried and did not know what to do. . . . Gamal arrived while I was in the bathroom. I washed my hands and went out to see him. It was so late, so I prepared the suhour [a pre-dawn meal eaten before a day of fasting], and ate with him. I must have looked worried because he asked me what was wrong with me. I replied, 'Nothing, I was just tired from working at the school all day and then the kids at home.' . . . He wanted another child so badly. He in fact wants two or three more children. I did not want to tell him about this problem because I did not know what was going to happen if he found out. . . . I had this problem for one week before I told any one. . . . I did not even tell my mother at first because I knew what her reaction was going to be. . . . I told one of my close friends at work.

Nawal, Amina's colleague, told her: "I do not think you should tell Gamal yet, he will think again that this is an excuse for not keeping this child or not having another one . . . but I think you must go to the doctor."

Nawal is a year older than Amina. She is married to a civil engineer working for the Cairo's city council. She was born in Cairo and has two sons aged four and six. Her deceased parents were originally from Minya, in central Egypt. Her father was an agriculture engineer and her mother a housewife. Amina confided to Nawal that she was completely distressed about this event. Her distress was not only because this was her first time facing such a problem, but because she thought she had no one to talk to about it. Amina said that if it were not for Nawal, who insisted on knowing why Amina was as pale as a "white sheet of cotton cloth" (*zayy al-bafta al-beda*), she would have never offered the information voluntarily. Amina was also confused because

> my heart knew what the action of my husband was going to be
> if I had told him; he'll think I don't want any children from him.
> Also I knew the reaction of my mother . . . I did not want to
> create a problem from nothing. . . . My mother never liked my
> husband. She thinks he is using me like a a cooking pot
> (*ma'un*), just to have children . . . she thinks he does this to
> compensate for the difference of his economic status and his
> family's, relative to my family's (*wad'uh al-iqtisadi huwwa wi 'iltuh
> bi-l-nisba li-'ilti*). . . . She told me many times in front
> of him and behind his back to be careful with my 'body and
> health.'

However, after six weeks of doctor shopping with Nawal, using multiple excuses to leave work early or leave home for such purposes, it was found out that Amina probably had a benign fibroma in the uterine wall. The more the fetus grew, the more pressure there would be on this fibrous tumor, the more bleeding, and the greater the danger to her uterus. During her fifth month of pregnancy, Amina was faced with the choice of termination of pregnancy or continuation at her own risk, and she was also faced with the inescapable task of telling her family.

Social Relations and Illness Practice

Both Amina and Ayman come from what has been traditionally known in Egypt as 'middle-class' families. Or in other words they both come from the bourgeoisie of Egypt, whose education has accorded them a social status based on their distance from manual labor and their proximity to intellectual labor and access to supplementary economic capital. In both cases, there is a perceived and actual dichotomy between their class affiliation and other lower classes. For both, their class affiliation inculcated in them the parameters of their experience and corporal expression—they had a subculture. In the case of illness practice, class loyalty became evident in their re-erecting the boundaries between the self as educated bourgeoisie and the perceived 'other' as a homogenous (relatively) lower class.

In both cases, a certain condition took over and became their life-world. In both cases this common feature resulted in a heightened interaction with multiple players. Notwithstanding gender differences, their class subculture became a frame of references, a scale on which perceptions and actions are evaluated. As members of a certain class, their identity was created, where perceptions and actions became the outward manifestation to reaffirm—albeit not always—a person's place in society and a society's place in the individual.[8]

Affiliation and Practice

Being a member of a certain class in Egypt accords the person a subculture, which in turn grants at least two fundamental properties: a social network that matches the needs and resources required to maintain one's place in his/her class habitus, and a certain code of experiential knowledge and corporeality one employs in different social settings and encounters, including illness practice.

Illness practice, then, is a social phenomenon, an embodiment of personal affiliations to kin, gender, and class habitus. Systems of culture, politics, and economics are intertwined to reproduce prevailing forms of social differentiation, which in turn create their own subsystems of social and illness practice. While state-sponsored healthcare in the 1950s and 1960s gave the impression that all people are born with equal

---

8. This is not a recent phenomenon. The domain of disease and illness has always been a domain for practice of class maintenance in Egypt. For example, Gallagher notes that even though public service was in the minds of upper-class Egyptian women during public health crises, this cannot—and should not—be separated from their class interests (Gallagher 1990: 54). For the upper classes, their notion of public service in cases of diseases and illnesses is rooted in their interest to maintain their class habitus.

access to healthcare in Egypt, current shortage of funding and maldistribution in healthcare give the impression that *fi nas wi fi nas* is the rule, as can be seen in the examples cited. Ayman said:

> I was too embarrassed to ask for a referral to go to the doctor
> of the camp or the military hospital. . . . I knew I needed to go
> there in order to be allowed a leave, but I could not get myself
> to ask for that. . . . I could not go there because this means
> that I trust a doctor working in this place to diagnose my
> condition. . . . This would mean that I cannot afford to go to
> a better private doctor. . . . It is only the poor who go to this
> kind of doctor. . . . Of all those who are doing their military
> service on the camp, it is those who cannot afford a private
> doctor or who need an excuse to go on a leave that go to this
> doctor. . . . All of 'us' don't really like to go there. . . . 'We' are
> the educated people who come from Cairo or other cities . . .
> We come from educated families. Some of us have parents who
> are teachers, doctors, general managers, own businesses, etc.

Ayman's comments open doors on at least two interesting additions to his story, as to who are 'us' and about what his condition is? In other words, 'we' are the offspring of the bourgeoisie created largely by the regime of the 1950s and 1960s. Ayman and Amina are members of a social class produced by and predicated on the modernization agenda of the post-revolution state in Egypt, confirming Marx's view that history and social structure change on the basis of a connection between classes and states (Knapp 1994: 50). However, ironically, the bourgeoisie of the 1960s mutated itself in replacing the old bourgeoisie; so instead of dissolving disparities between classes, disparities intensified and class conflict gained momentum (Siam 1995: 134; Zaalouk 1989). In the 1990s, this class is part of yet another class conflict associated with market economics (Gad 1994; Siam 1995; Zaalouk 1989). In all cases, the ammunition in the class conflict is cultural, social, material, and symbolic capital. The manifestation is in social and illness practice.

The case of Ayman and his group stands in sharp contrast to other bourgeois and proletariat. Fitting into a majority, he and others see no need to be concerned too much with others below them, since the others are *nas baladi wi fellahin* (traditional people and peasants) or *mustawahum mutawadi'* (of humble standards). His group seems unwittingly, or not, to hold more esteem for those higher than their class, copying them in belief and action.

Amina's view, with her similar class affiliation, does not depart too far from Ayman's: "Of course I did not mention or ask anyone else from my work for advice on my problem. . . . This is not something one talks about with [women] work colleagues. . . . Also most of them are *baladi*, coming from a humble standard *(mustawa mutawad')*."

Amina could not talk to her husband and mother for fear of their impositions on her biological, moral, and even social life. In contrast to Ayman, whose experience was shaped without much questioning from his part, Amina was more cautious. This is probably because she has been bluntly subjected to similar incidents at other times, or because her condition is related to matters of reproduction, a sensitive matter in every family in Egypt, or perhaps because she is feistier than Ayman. It is not easy to pinpoint the importance of each factor in such complex situations.

But on the other hand, she could not share her problem except with one friend at work who fitted the class classification perceived to be capable of understanding and appreciating such a biological condition. Her scant material capital was being rapidly depleted by the demands of weeks of private medical care, leaving her with only the cultural and social capital available in the subculture, which she had to resort to later.

The logic of social and illness practice is one of class ascription and is maintained through classism. Everyone has a class—of a sort—and everyone is put in his/her appropriate class category and its subculture. Identification of the logic of class affiliation is helpful in all aspects of life: in seeking a job, a spouse, an investment, an education, and healthcare. Classism and class disparity can be employed to rationalize and justify, *inter alia*, being refused a job or getting it, being treated disrespectfully or respectfully at health services, being refused or accepted at private schools, getting along with neighbors or not, getting a fair deal in life or not. Affiliation in Egypt then is not only familial. Class consciousness and class loyalty are just as strong predictors of access to resources, social action, and illness practice.

Class Infusion in the Patient-Doctor Encounter

Ayman seemed more worried about keeping his problem unnoticed by others than about the problem itself. Ayman's main problem was not that his physical condition was gradually taking a strong hold on his thinking, it was rather how to negotiate his place in his class habitus in life and the medical establishment now that his health had been altered.

Mahmoud, his friend proved to be a good helper. "Mahmoud told me that I should tell the doctor everything," Ayman said. "Tell him exactly when my condition started (and) how it progressed from one step to the other. . . . I should pay attention to appear concerned, otherwise he (the doctor) would think I am there just to get him to recommend a vacation for me or something."

Mahmoud's advice was reaffirmed by Ayman's mother, whose concern went beyond showing rationality, towards bodily hexis (Bourdieu 1977), which connotes manners, movement, and body presentation. "Of course, when he [the doctor] saw how he [Ayman] was dressed, acted and spoke," recounted Ayman's mother, "he realized he came from a respectable family ('ailah mohtaramah), and was treated respectfully . . . and with more attention."

Ayman, on his own, prepared himself for his medical encounters by being clean, shaven, dressed in a pair of dressy trousers and an ironed shirt, and wearing some nice cologne. He could not explain why he made such an effort, except in terms of relating this interaction to other events he considered significant, for which he would always prepare and dress in a way that would make him look 'respectable.'

Amina's preparation for her pre-clinical encounter included much of the same rationality and aesthetics. Her repertoire, additionally, included some English words, which she used in her medical encounter. Words such as 'bleeding,' and 'weakness' were used to indicate at once Amina's place on the social ladder and her place on the illness ladder. She was not told by anyone to use certain vocabulary but 'felt' this should give the doctors a good indication of her educational and social standing, or in other words her economic, social, and cultural capital.

Indeed, with the help of Nawal, she became more versed in the lingo of her condition. Whenever she had to go for another test or to another doctor, she integrated more of her newly acquired medical vocabulary in each encounter. This was now elevated to talking about 'anaemia,' 'fibroma,' 'ultrasonography,' and 'oedema.' The language of the encounter reflected her embracing the medical categorization of her condition. But, more significantly, the idioms associated with her medical categorization and the idioms of her class mutually reinforced each other. With the combination of medical knowledge and her class habitus, she constructed the logic of her illness practice as an experiential process.

It is difficult to know to what extent Ayman and Amina's self-representation influenced the outcome of their clinical encounters. But, their commonly shared perception and their illness practice influenced their interaction with the medical system and doctors, and provided them with clues as to the quality of and satisfaction with their encounter. Hence, the logic of medical encounters is located within the dialectics of class subculture in Egypt. Ayman may have been advised to dress in a certain way, but he was not directly advised to dress in certain colors or certain designs or a certain combination of colors—which he did in order to look 'decent' and 'middle class.'

Amina, on the other hand, was never told to sprinkle her medical encounters with English words, but did so partially consciously, partly unwittingly. Her language and body comport were contained by the physical space of the clinic and power relations in the clinical setting. However, she embodied the cultural values, gender, and class relations whose boundaries were less visible and more pervasive than her family affiliation only. Her condition, logically, followed the seams of her identity as a mother, wife, and obliging daughter, but her language was her own way of creating a space just for her. She noted that, if nothing else, at least her vocabulary helped her overcome her embarrassment about her condition as a middle-class Egyptian woman revealing her body and its dysfunctions to others. It is her subculture through which her bodily dysfunctions were experienced and practiced.

Consequently, it is possible to conclude that illness practice, of which the doctor-patient relationship is an element, is predicated on forms of culturally available capital and the inculcated ways to manage this capital. Access to and value of this capital are at times subdued and covert, and at times overt and explicit, or more complex still, they usually occur as a mixture of social practice as can be seen in the case of aesthetics in illness practice.

The Aesthetics of Illness Practice

Health and illness perception and practice are unquestionably class- and subculture-linked. Ayman often represents his taste in clothing, scent, popular cultural expression, and facial appearance in much the same way as he represents his choice of healthcare services or conduct in medical encounters. These, perceptually and practically, distinguish him from 'others.' A class subculture is therefore complex.

Illness practice relies on culturally salient stimuli and sensory paths of distinction. Ayman, in his illness practice, perceives the relative value of particular sensory stimuli through the filters of his class habitus. For example, he preferred—in accordance with members of his social network—to go to a private doctor for his condition. Ayman's reasons, beyond perceived technical competence, included perceptual elements that are temporal: "I don't have time in the morning to go to a government hospital where the outpatient clinic operates only until 11:00 A.M."; spatial: "Private doctors are better because one gets a reasonable seat in a waiting room with better lights"; auditory: "One never hears the nurses or aides screaming at each other or at patients. There is also more privacy when you speak to the doctor"; olfactory: "One is less likely to smell garbage or stinking toilets"; and tactile: "One is going to sit in a comfortable upholstered, or at least cushioned, and clean chair, not a wooden bench. . . . One does not have to touch filthy examination tables or partition screens." Ayman's sensory experience is infused with the dynamics that articulate his class habitus. This confirms that body experience is always engaged in the "dynamic distribution of power" (Crawford 1984: 95). Illness practice, then, is not a natural but a naturalized cultural phenomenon.

In the Egyptian context aesthetics is therefore largely a matter of differentiated access to capital. Material capital and cultural capital "cannot function as capital until . . . inserted into the objective relations between the system . . . and the system producing the producers" (Bourdieu 1977: 186). It follows logically that practice, which is capital dependent, acquires its meaning from being inserted into a value system that reproduces its sources. If particularities of illness practice—such as in aesthetics—do not have the potential to be inserted in a value system that is culturally reproducible, they would probably be abandoned.

Illness Practice and Life Course

The narrative of social distinction between self and others, tradition and modernity is evident in the situations where Ayman acts according to his (national) class subculture: "I am not like the sons of low-class people and the peasants (*ana mish zayy awlad al-nas al-baladi wa-l-fallahin*)." In other instances he is less direct: "I am not like the others (*ana mish zayy al-tanyin*)." In all cases, the exclusivity of the class to which Ayman and Amina belong is only justifiable based on their own perceived notions of themselves as superior. There is no denial that there are some objective grounds on which social distinctions and subcultural heterogeneity are perceived. The point is that "life choices are not randomly distributed" and that in illness, as in life, "choices do not merely co-occur: each helps to determine the other" (Young 1982: 261).

Class Subculture Illness and Time

In itself, the study of economic modes of production and capital accumulation does not lead us onto a natural path of knowing about people's experience in health and illness (Doyal 1995; Doyal and Pennel 1979). Stories like those of Ayman and Amina can help us understand more of how class subculture dynamics influence some seemingly banal aspects of illness practice. The perceptions of Amina, Ayman, and their network represent a local knowledge of essential social practice. In these perceptions 'others' are constructed in ways that conveniently maintain the self's relatively advantageous position in social interaction, even in illness. Perceptions of different classes are similar in that the construction of the 'other' is based on a host of cultural, economic, and ideological factors of which aesthetics and illness practice are only a manifestation of the perceptual foundation of the 'place' of self and other in society. This occurs, even, or maybe especially, at times when the person's physical capital is under threat. Class habitus and management of capital take on prominent dimensions at times of economic or health crisis. At those times, self may become too narrowly defined:

> [I]nteraction and communication inside each stratum become
> more intensified and deepened than interaction with other strata.
> [Thus] the person who belongs to lower strata is less
> courageous in dealing with higher strata, as the latter become
> more closed onto themselves, *practicing rituals that can build around*
> *them a wall of arrogance and disdain for anything that is lower* (Zayed
> 1990: 162, author's translation and emphasis).

The trajectories of the Aymans and Aminas in illness practice and social practice could be a natural response to assaults of rapid changes in the economic and subsequent cultural configuration of society (see Bourdieu 1984: 111–112). This may explain the internal fissures within social categories and class habitus. Where change from without is strong, intra-class habitus loyalties come under attack. The private world of a class habitus can then turn into private worlds of subcultures within a class habitus. With sustained assault from without, the conditions for a subculture become more instituted.

To summarize the intricacy of the relationship between culture, class, and interaction with state apparatus, Ahmed Zayed explains:

Thus the private world of each social group becomes a safer world . . . extraneous modernization process, which affected the social structure has not changed completely the concepts of affiliation to family, extended family, and region. In this light, class structure does not allow communication, as modernity has not removed all elements separating people. In light of these circumstances, we expect the person to be more trusting of his [her] relatives, those from his village or city. . . . The matter could go as far as excessive subjectivism when we find the person entwined around his family or himself only . . . subsequently *self becomes the center of the world.* (Zayed 1990: 163, author's translation and emphasis)

Ayman and Amina's perceptions transcend their gender differences. Their class is not only different from others, they perceive themselves as superior to others. This superiority is partially attributed to their direct and indirect socioeconomic status, but more importantly it is attributed to their moral or symbolic capital made available through their class habitus. According to Bourdieu, "secondary properties" are at least equally influential in determining class habitus (Bourdieu 1984: 102). Accordingly, Ayman and Amina are inculcated with the material and the ideological privilege/properties of their class: they are better, more knowledgeable, and more secure in their feelings and perceptions. They have 'class,' even, or especially, when they fall ill. Ironically, this is continually being reaffirmed because it is continually being challenged.

Class hierarchy is held together by the "unproductive uses of economic surplus" (Eyer 1984: 52). In Egypt, class hierarchy is also held together by the surplus of other capital: symbolic, social, and cultural. While economic surplus is usually used to maintain inter-class hierarchy, Amina and Ayman are also engaged in maintaining intra-class hierarchy. For Ayman and Amina, an opportune time to emphasize intra-class hierarchy is when their physical capital is being compromised. Clearly what transpires is the presence of specific intra-class strategies of employing surplus capital, in its complex combination, to maintain social class hierarchy. Hence, the ethos of illness practice is not to regain control and overcome "somatic vulnerability" (see Crawford 1984: 74). Rather, it is to regain control of the situated self. It is not about getting well but about getting even. Just as health is associated with a moral discourse (76), illness practice is associated with a political discourse. In this discourse, knowledge follows power, both of which are individually experienced and culturally produced.

Conclusions: Illness Designations and the Nuances of Culture

Class habitus plays an important role in illness practice, including disclosure and choice of timing and place of healthcare. While to a great extent the condition itself dictates how malleable a person becomes in seeking and accepting advice (see Inhorn 1994), in Egypt, one cannot just share bodily dysfunctions without being loyal to class habitus affiliation. It has been argued here that understanding the subcultures of social classes is the first step toward a thorough understanding of illness practice. The term intentionally implies less rationality than illness management, illness behavior (see Richman 1987), or sickness career (Twaddle 1981). More than Talcott Parson's 'sick role,' which "as an 'ideal type,' [lacks] spatio-temporal and cultural dimensions [and] has obvious limitations as an empirical referent" (Richman 1987: 77), illness practice is more accommodating of the context of class habitus within which it takes shape.

It is imperative that we study the historical roots of people's perceptions and practice at times of health and illness. As we have seen here, not only do people rely on their existential experiences to deal with illnesses, their physical and material world systematically influences their perceptual world as well. It is to be hoped that this study will make a significant contribution in our understanding of social and healthcare needs, and the systematic inequality underlying those needs. To refine the definition that was proposed earlier in this chapter, illness practice has been used here to imply historically-rooted, consensual, cultural knowledge and actions produced through an interactive process between culturally constructed conscious and subconscious inculcations of values and meanings. These values are shaped by disparities in economic, social, cultural, physical, and symbolic capital. It is embedded in a subculture predicated on a class habitus, which is—as is illness practice—always transient and dynamic. This concept opens the door for more sophisticated studies of social class, culture, and illness in Egypt and the Arab world.

Postscript

Ayman was treated for six months with different analgesics and unspecified 'nerve strengthening medications,' by different private doctors. He never went to see the 'Red Sea' doctor. He was later diagnosed with a chronic depressive disorder for which he is under treatment. Amina indeed finally told her husband, who went to the doctor with her, before the two of them together told her mother, and before she finally went through a traumatic medical abortion. Amina confides that neither her body nor her life has been the same since then.

Bibliography

Abu-Lughod, Janet L., 1971, *Cairo, 1001 Years of the City Victorious*. Princeton: Princeton University Press.

Abu-Lughod, Lila, 1986, *Veiled Sentiments: Honor and Poetry in a Bedouin Society*. Berkeley: University of California Press.

Barakat, Halim, ed., 1985, *Contemporary North Africa: Issues of Development and Integration*. London: Croom Helm.

Bhabha, Homi, 1990a, "Narrating the Nation," *Nation and Narration*, H. Bhabha, ed. London: Routledge.

————, 1990b, "The Third Space: Interview with Homi Bhabha," *Identity: Community, Culture, Difference*, Jonathan Rutherford, ed. London: Lawrence and Wishart.

Blane, David, 1982, "Inequality and Social Class," *Sociology as Applied to Medicine*, Donald L. Patrick and Graham Scambler, eds. London: Bailliere Tindall.

Bourdieu, Pierre, 1977, *Outline of a Theory of Practice*. Cambridge: Cambridge University Press.

————, 1984, *Distinction: A Social Critique of the Judgement of Taste*. Cambridge: Harvard University Press.

————, 1990, *The Logic of Practice*. Stanford: Stanford University Press.

Burkitt, Ian, 1991, "Social Selves: Theories of the Social Formation of Personality," *Current Sociology*, 39 (3): 1–227.

Calhoun, Craig, 1993, "Habitus, Field, and Capital: The Question of Historical Specificity," *Bourdieu: Critical Perspectives*, Craig Calhoun, Edward LiPuma, and Moishe Postone, eds. Chicago: The University of Chicago Press.

Crawford, Robert, 1984, "A Cultural Account of 'Health': Control, Release, and the Social Body," *Issues in the Political Economy of Health Care*, John B. McKinlay, ed. New York: Tavistock Publications.

Dessouki, Ali E. Hillal, 1982, "The Politics of Income Distribution in Egypt," *The Political Economy of Income Distribution in Egypt*, Gouda Abdel-Khalek and Robert Tignor, eds. New York: Holmes & Meier Publishers.

Doyal, Lesley, 1995, *What Makes Women Sick: Gender and the Political Economy of Health*. New Brunswick: Rutgers University Press.

Doyal, Lesley and Imogen Pennell, 1979, *The Political Economy of Health*. London: Pluto Press.

Early, Evelyn, 1993, *Baladi Women of Cairo: Playing with an Egg and a Stone*. Boulder: Lynne Rienner Publishers.

Eyer, Joe, 1984, "Capitalism, Health, and Illness," *Issues in the Political Economy of Health Care*, John B. McKinlay, ed. New York: Tavistock Publications.

Fergani, Nader, 1994, "On the Distribution of Social Position in Egypt with Particular Reference to Gender Differentials," *al-Majalla al-ijtima'iya al-qawmiya*, 31 (1): 229–244.

Gad, Mahmoud, 1994, *al-Tarkib al-tabaqi li-l-madina al-misriya fi-l-'asr al-hadith*. Cairo: Maktabat al-Nahda al-Misriya.

———, 1995a, Upper Class in an Upper Egypt City *(al-Tabaqa al-'ulya fi ihda mudun al-Sa'id)*. Cairo: Dar al-Fikr al-Hadith.

———, 1995b, *al-Tabaqa al-wusta al-misriya*. Cairo: Dar al-Thaqafa al-Jadida.

Gallagher, Nancy Elizabeth, 1990, *Egypt's Other Wars: Epidemics and the Politics of Public Health*. Cairo: The American University in Cairo Press.

Good, Byron J., 1994, *Medicine, Rationality, and Experience: An Anthropological Perspective*. Cambridge: Cambridge University Press.

Good, Mary-Jo Delvecchio and Byron J. Good, 1982, "Patient Requests in Primary Care Clinics," *Clinically Applied Anthropology: Anthropologists in Health Science Settings*, Noel J. Chrisman and Thomas W. Maretzki, eds. Dordrecht: D. Reidel Publishing Company.

Hahn, Robert, 1995, *Sickness and Healing: An Anthropological Perspective*. New Haven: Yale University Press.

Ibrahim, Saad Eddin, 1982, "Social Mobility and Income Distribution in Egypt, 1952–1977," *The Political Economy of Income Distribution in Egypt*, Gouda Abdel-Khaled and Robert Tignor, eds. New York: Holmes & Meier Publishers.

Imam, Samia Saeed, 1991, *Man yamluk Misr? Dirasa tahliliya li-l-usil al-ijtima'iya li-nukhbat al-infitah al-iqtisadi fi-l-mujtama' al-misri: 1974–1980.* Damascus: IBAL Publishing.

Inhorn, Marcia C., 1994, *Quest for Conception: Gender, Infertility, and Egyptian Medical Traditions.* Philadelphia: University of Pennsylvania Press.

Katon, Wayne and Arthur Kleinman, 1981, "Doctor-Patient Negotiation and Other Social Science Strategies in Patient Care," *The Relevance of Social Sciences for Medicine.* Leon Eisenberg and Arthur Kleinman, eds. Dordrecht: Kluwer Academic Publishers.

Kleinman, Arthur, Paul E. Brodwin, Byron J. Good, Mary-Jo DelVecchio Good, 1994, "Pain as Human Experience: An Introduction," *Pain as Human Experience: An Anthropological Perspective*, Mary-Jo DelVecchio Good, Paul E. Brodwin, Byron J. Good, and Arthur Kleinman, eds. Berkeley: University of California Press.

Knapp, Peter, 1994, *One World–Many Worlds: Contemporary Sociological Theory.* New York: Harper Collins.

Kuhnke, Laverne, 1990, *Lives at Risk. Public Health in Nineteenth-Century Egypt.* Cairo: The American University in Cairo Press.

Marsot, Afaf Lutfi al-Sayyid, 1984, *Egypt in the Reign of Muhammad Ali.* Cambridge: Cambridge University Press.

Marx, Karl, and Fredrick Engels, 1971, "The Communist Manifesto," *Essential Works of Marxism*, Arthur Mandel, ed. New York: Bantam Books.

El Missiri Nadim, Nawal, 1975, "The Relationships Between the Sexes in a Harah of Cairo," Ph.D. Thesis, Department of Anthropology, Indiana University.

———, 1985, "Family Relationships in a Harah in Cairo," *Arab Society: Social Science Perspectives*, Nicholas S. Hopkins and Saad Eddin Ibrahim, eds. Cairo: The American University in Cairo Press.

Moore, Henrietta L., 1996, *Space, Text, and Gender: An Anthropological Study of the Marakwet of Kenya.* New York: The Guilford Press.

Morgan, Myfanway, Michael Calnan, and Nick Manning, 1985, *Sociological Approaches to Health and Medicine.* London: Croom Helm.

Morsy, Soheir A., 1993, *Gender, Sickness, and Healing in Rural Egypt: Ethnography in Historical Context.* Boulder: Westview Press.

Noweer, Abdel Salam, 1994, "al-hirak al-ijtima'iy wa-l-taghyir al-siyasi fi Misr" *al-Majalla al-ijtima'iya al-qawmiya*, 31 (1): 209–228.

Obeyesekere, Gananath, 1990, *The Work of Culture: Symbolic Transformation in Psychoanalysis and Anthropology.* Chicago: The University of Chicago Press.

Parsons, Talcott, 1951, *The Social System.* Glencoe: Free Press.

Patai, Raphael, 1973, *The Arab Mind*. New York: Charles Scribner's Sons.
Postone, Moishe, Edward LiPuma, and Craig Calhoun, 1993, "Introduction: Bourdieu and Social Theory," *Bourdieu: Critical Perspectives*, Craig Calhoun, Edward LiPuma, and Moishe Postone, eds. Chicago: The University of Chicago Press.
Richman, J., 1987, *Medicine and Health*. London: Longman.
Rugh, Andrea B., 1984, *Family in Contemporary Egypt*. Cairo: The American University in Cairo Press.
Sachs, Lisbeth, 1989, "Misunderstanding as Therapy: Doctors, Patients and Medicines in a Rural Clinic in Sri Lanka," *Culture, Medicine and Psychiatry*, 13 (3): 335–349.
Siam, Shehata, 1995, *al dawlah wi i'adet intaj il faqr*. Cairo: Ramatan.
Singer, Merril, 1987, "Cure, Care, and Control: An Ectopic Encounter with Biomedical Obstetrics," *Encounters with Biomedicine: Case Studies in Medical Anthropology*. Hans A. Baer, ed. New York: Gordon and Breach Science Publishers.
Tignor, Robert, 1982, "Equity in Egypt's Recent Past: 1945–1952," *The Political Economy of Income Distribution in Egypt*, Gouda Abdel-Khaled and Robert Tignor, eds. New York: Holmes & Meier Publishers.
Tucker, Judith E, 1993, "The Arab Family in History: 'Otherness' and the Study of the Family," *Arab Women: Old Boundaries, New Frontiers*, Judith E. Tucker, ed. Indianapolis: Indiana University Press.
Twaddle, Andrew, 1981, "Sickness and the Sickness Career: Some Implications," *The Relevance of Social Sciences for Medicine*, Leon Eisenberg and Arthur Kleinman, eds. Dordrecht: Kluwer Academic Publishers.
Wikan, Unni, 1996, *Tomorrow, God Willing: Self-Made Destinies in Cairo*. Chicago: The University of Chicago Press.
Wiles, Rose and Joan Higgins, 1996, "Doctor-Patient Relationships in the Private Sector: Patients' Perceptions," *Sociology of Health and Illness*, 18 (3): 341–356.
Williams, Simon J., 1995, "Theorising Class, Health, and Lifestyle: Can Bourdieu Help Us?" *Sociology of Health and Illness*, 17 (5): 577–604.
Young, Allan, 1982, "The Anthropologies of Illness and Sickness," *Annual Review of Anthropology*, 11: 257–285.
Zaalouk, Malak, 1989, *Power, Class and Foreign Capital in Egypt: The Rise of the New Bourgeoisie*. London: Zed Books.
Zayed, Ahmed, 1990, *al-Misry al-mu'asir: Muqaraba nazariya wa imbiriqiya li-ba'd ab'ad al-shakhsiya al-qawmiya al-misriya*. Cairo: National Center for Sociological and Criminological Research.

Mushahra

The Justice and Injustice of Infertility

HANIA SHOLKAMY

The Quest for Fertility

This chapter is about issues of female fertility and infertility among Upper Egyptians. The question that I am attempting to consider, dare I say, answer, is this: How have women tolerated, and how do they continue to tolerate and cope with the onerous pressure that is put upon them to be fertile and to produce healthy sons? Rather than launch into an epidemiological study of infertility, reproductive morbidity, or of rates of polygamy and divorce, I would like to convey an understanding of the context in which these pressures and responses are experienced.

I propose to do so by examining the gendered discourse of fertility and infertility as it is expressed in the belief in *mushahra*, an infertility spell. I suggest *mushahra* is not only a dynamic and potent belief but a mental and social construct that conveys some understanding of the daily life of women and men. Indeed, despite the profusion of work about Arab women in villages, towns, and those living in tribes, there is still room for the consideration of aspects of women's lives that contribute to the diversity, dynamics, and subtlety employed in their construction of the cultural contexts in which they live.

Arab women have been the objects of much critical scholarship in the past two decades (cf. Abu-Lughod 1989; Beck and Keddie 1978; Tucker 1993; Rassam 1980; Rosen 1989). In her highly illuminating review of 1989, Lila Abu-Lughod borrows Arjun Appadurai's concept of Zones of Theory to address representations of the Arab world in the field of English language anthropological writings. She mentions the study of Arab women as one zone or "dominant theoretical metonym," which she calls 'Harem Theory' and which dominates our theorizing about the Arab region to the exclusion of other concepts (Abu-Lughod 1989: 279, 287).

Theorizing about women has tended to be a question of reification and demystification. Stereotypical accounts of the lives and times of Arab women suffering under the yoke of gender inequality, segregation, and absence from centers of power and decision-making are typical of earlier work. These images survived only to be challenged by an oppositional stance that focused on the power women wield in the private sphere, the fluidity of the private and the public spheres, and the active roles that women assume in constructing the worlds in which they live (Abu-Lughod 1989). This ongoing evolution of the study of Arab women has tended to be characterized by a 'revelationary' tone. Writers, most of whom are women, tend to 'reveal' the true wisdom, wit, and wondrous will of the women about whom they write. There is an assertiveness and a conclusivity to this overwhelmingly affectionate genre of anthropology, which at times replicates the problematics of less gender-informed analysis.

With some notable exceptions (cf. Boddy 1989; Abu-Lughod 1993a, 1993b), scholars seem to be trading in what Maurice Bloch has called "post hoc rationalizations" of what women and their lives are like (Bloch 1991). Many of the accounts that have currency are problematic in that they present one interpretation per symbol, relationship, or event. Despite the wealth of ethnographic description and the depth of rapport, which few anthropologists fail to stress, some ethnographies still opt for gloss, taking for granted metonyms as shorthand for the daily life and the individuals about whom they write.

In this paper I shall consider ideas and principles that inform practices of individuals and groups when it comes to reproduction in an attempt to provide a textured, polysemous, less-than-conclusive understanding of some women and their fertility. Through the consideration of *mushahra*, which has wide currency in most parts of Egypt, and indeed in the rest of the Arab region, I shall attempt to elaborate on its practices and practitioners only to transcend the immediate function of such a belief, so as to ponder its significance as a local tool of analysis and exegesis that addresses probability, equality, and the construction of community. In considering *mushahra*, I hope to avoid the metonymic gloss of Harem Theory and to highlight this common and lived belief and its practice as a field of potential and possibility through which women, and also men, express their values and concerns.

I shall first present a brief explanation of what *mushahra* is and illustrate how its mention and practice imposed itself on my work. I would then like to review the literature that addresses *mushahra*, whether partially or fully, before going on to investigate the functions and structures of this belief and to elaborate on its significance in Upper Egypt.

The material that I shall use to approach this question is based upon fieldwork in a village/hamlet in the vicinity of Abnub in the governorate of Asyut approximately 400 kilometers south of Cairo. This hamlet lies to the southeast of Asyut city on what is by and large recently reclaimed agricultural land. The villagers among whom I lived are Arab Muslims. By Arab I am referring to their Bedouin origins. They are descendants of settlers who came from the clan of Matir who are a part of the tribe of Arab al-A'sar. The village is small by Egyptian standards. It has a population of approximately 2,000 people who live on a land area of eight feddans (a feddan equals 4,200 square meters), which forms the nucleated settlement area, excluding farmland. The inhabitants work in agriculture but many are migrant laborers in Saudi Arabia, Jordan, Libya, Cairo, and in the Suez Canal zone.

There are no women in the village employed in anything other than household and agricultural work. There are a couple of seamstresses and healer/midwives. Among the generation of women, who are now in their late teens and early twenties, there are some girls who have finished their high school diplomas but as yet none have taken the plunge into the labor market.

This village is poor relative to other parts of Asyut but is no more isolated or incorporated than any other Egyptian village. While it is on the remote fringes of the fertile Nile valley, its high degree of outward labor migration has brought inhabitants in contact with urban Egypt and with communities in the Gulf. I mention this to dispel any notion of *mushahra* as being a local survival of times gone by and specific only to this village or area.

The paramount importance of children, particularly boys, has often been commented on and has come to form an uncontested orthodoxy in the ethnographic, feminist, and literary writings on rural Upper Egypt (Blackmen 1927; Ayrout 1963; Morsy 1993). On the other hand, infertility, whether temporary or permanent, is a reality no community can escape. In one 17-country WHO study conducted in the early 1990s, 27 percent of the infertile couples in the sample were infertile due to no demonstrable causes (Mascie-Taylor 1993: 43). Writing in 1927

Winifred Blackman remarks, "The fact that so many methods of curing barrenness are employed by the peasant is an indication that, despite the high birthrate, infertility in women is not uncommon in Egypt." (Blackman 1927: 108). Indeed, despite the staunchly antinatalist policy of the government and the alarmingly high fertility rate in rural Upper Egypt, where the fertility rate is 6.7 births per woman (CAPMAS 1993: 147), the reported level of primary sterility is 2.7 percent in Egypt on the whole and infertility is very much part of the reality and concern of men and women in Upper Egypt (126).

The responses of Muslim men to female infertility, as far as the literature is concerned, can be summarized in two words: divorce and polygamy (Boddy 1989: 114). This is a gross generalization but one that has been overstressed by analysts and writers. But what about women? How do they respond to the uncertainty that haunts every new bride, and to the quest for the essential title of *Umm fulan* (the mother of so-and-so) and the possibility of never attaining this most prized and respected of titles?

Mushahra provides an explanation and toleration for slow pregnancy and female infertility. According to the Dictionary of Egyptian Arabic, *mushahra* is "To put a spell of barrenness on a woman by entering into her presence during the daytime of the forty day period after her giving birth, carrying, e.g., jewels, fresh meat, or the first fruits of the season" (Hinds and Badawi 1986).

Mushahra is a spell that is believed to afflict girls and women by making them infertile or by affecting the milk supply of feeding mothers. It can also, by extension, affect the young child of the afflicted woman. The word *mushahra* is a conjugation of the Arabic word for month *(shahr)*. Literally *mushahra* means 'monthing.'

Girls and woman who are going through rites of passage, which lead to life-cycle transformations and involve the loss of blood or the production of milk are considered to be in a state of sacred vulnerability, from the moment they experience these rites until the birth of the new moon, which signals the end of their susceptibility. Life-cycle transformations which thus jeopardize a woman's well-being are circumcision, defloration and marriage, child birth, weaning, and miscarriage.

If during her period of vulnerability a girl or woman is entered upon by one who is also in jeopardy, they may cause each other *mushahra*. More likely, however, the female in confinement suffers, not the one who enters. Blood and death can cause *mushahra*, so can the extension and some symbolic representations of both. Black eggplant brought into a room where there is a vulnerable girl or woman can cause *mushahra*. Abd al-Rahman Ismail writing in 1892 says that indigo dye was believed to have the same affect. Both eggplants and indigo are black and are considered to be symbolic representations of death. Moreover, eggplants are in some contexts considered symbolic representations of the placenta (Boddy 1989: 104–5). Raw meat bears similar potency. The fresh blood that meat contains is deemed to be the active ingredient. Visitors coming straight from the cemetery can also afflict a woman. This is death by proxy that brings about the spell. Likewise, people coming from the market, where fresh blood flows from weekly slaughters, are dangerous for the same reason.

The elaborations on *mushahra*-inducing agents are infinite and are prescribed by the local environment of women. Whereas Marcia Inhorn writing about Alexandrian women says cats who have delivered or lost their young (involuntary weaning) can affect *mushahra*, in Upper Egypt dogs and donkeys are thought to possess the same capability (Inhorn 1994). There are no cats in the village where I did my fieldwork.

Mushahra-inducing persons and objects and their surrogates or substances are the self-same substances and agents that can revoke the spell. *Mushahra* is deflected by a repeat interaction with the self-same substances. Instead of continuing with this generic description I would like to refer to my field experiences to illustrate how mushahra works.

During the course of my fieldwork I could not avoid *mushahra*. Fertility per se was not a topic that I brought up, but my own fertility was the subject of much concern and seemed to impose itself due to the popular demand of my informants. In brief, I was considered perhaps to be afflicted with *mushahra* and as such became privy to the experiences of others who had themselves somehow caused, cured, or suffered from the spell. The following are a few summary excerpts from these conversations.

Our neighbor's daughter and I were circumcised together. We both wore *mashahir* (five or seven palm reeds knotted together) and we became well. Then she got married years ago and she waited for a child. She waited and waited but she could not get one. She saw a doctor but did not have the tests. My mother told her that she might be *mushohra* (afflicted with *mushahra*) since the time we were both circumcised. So I went over to her house and I peed on her pee and she took a bit of cloth and dipped it in the puddle and she wore it and a year later she had a boy. (Fayza, a girl in her late teens or early twenties, the eldest of eight siblings)

I thought that I would not get pregnant again. When I was weaning Atef I asked my niece Ola to enter the room. She was just circumcised and still wearing her *mashahir*. I know that it could have harmed Atef but I was careful and did not let her get close to him. But now I am carrying again. I think maybe the *mushahra* was undone by a donkey parted from her foal, or by one of the dogs. The dog in our neighbor's fields had a litter and they kept one apart from the mother so that they could use it to undo their own daughter's *mushahra*. Maybe this bitch crossed my path. Who knows? It could be many things. Before, when I had *mushahra* and wanted children, my aunt made me a *kabsa* (a mixture of vegetable peel, grains, and food stuffs mixed with the blood of a newly slaughtered animal and tied up in a piece of cloth) from the market. She told me to wear it but it was too big so I slept on it then on the first Friday of the new month I bathed in its water and I was cured. (Aziza, a woman in her late twenties and the mother of five children)

These women are so embarrassing. A neighbor's son got shot in a feud. There he was lying bleeding and dying at the edge of the fields. The person who did it was running, some women were screaming, and what does my (third) wife do? While running out screaming as if to accommodate the feelings of the dead man's family, she hurries out to step across the corpse. Our women believe that this helps them carry (children). Don't you think this is an embarrassment? Everyone knew what she was doing and there she was pretending to be crying when all she could think about was herself. Well, after that I gave her a good beating. Then after a while I went out to the desert to get her a local lizard, which is so quick and difficult to catch, but we know how to hunt for it. This lizard looks exactly like a scared man! When you get it and slaughter it looks like a human corpse, then women can cross over it and it has the same effect. (Abu Hussein, a man in his early forties and the father of twelve children, all from his third wife)

"The railroads are best, imagine how many people have died on the tracks," said the daughter. She herself had suffered from *mushahra*. She had cracked it by going to the *hasaniya* (the place in the mosque where the dead are washed and prepared for burial) and had gone round the stone slab three times during the Friday prayers and then she was cured. "No," said the mother. "There is nothing like the milk of a bitch parted from her little ones. I was *mushahra* many times. I used to make a doll with some of this milk and some flour and step over it. Then I would dissolve it in water and bathe with it on a Friday during afternoon prayers. (Hosn, a woman in her early thirties and the mother of five, discussing *mushahra* with her mother as they wait in a private physician's waiting room)

The above quotes exemplify a fraction of the ways by which one can enact or resolve *mushahra*. They also relay an important aspect of this spell—that is, its pervasiveness. I do not know of one woman in the village who did not voice an experience or opinion about the issue. More often than not, the topic would be brought up the following way: I would be visiting a woman I did not know, in the company of another who was close to her, usually the wife of my host. I would be asked if I had children and when a sad 'no' came, usually from my companion, the immediate very empathetic response would be, "Walk her through the eggplants," or "Is she using something?" The something being contraception. In this way the topic would be brought up, followed by optimistic promises for all kinds of cures.

In this way, I also began to notice and realize the unsaid features of the spell. Palm reeds and henna are characteristic of circumcisions and weddings. Both are powerful prophylactics. Recently circumcised girls, as mentioned, wear palm reeds to protect themselves and those they meet during their period of vulnerability. At any circumcision one can notice all the well-wishers wearing henna on their hands, as do the close family and friends at weddings. Henna is perhaps a proxy for blood. A groom wears henna so that he does not inadvertently cause his bride to be infertile and a bride wears henna so that she does not also inadvertently cause the groom to be infertile. This blood look-alike creates a false *mushahra*, which deflects the effect of real blood.

To partake in this belief does not preclude resort to biomedicine. When a woman has sought help in the clinic and the hospital, she is advised to remember if the 'cause' of her problem is *mushahra*. In that case she pursues both courses of therapy hoping to hit on the correct cause and so come up with the efficacious cure. Sometimes one course is pursued until there is enough money for the other. The case of Nagat illustrates this point. She and I had been going to see a healer in a village about 10 kilometers away from Abnub. I went for academic reasons and she for medical ones. Nagat has two children, aged seven and five. Her husband works in Saudi Arabia but comes home nearly every year. Despite these relatively frequent visits, she has been unable to become pregnant again. She is keen on more children although she does have a son. As we were waiting for a lift off the main road after our third visit to the healer, Nagat said: "If only I had the money to go see a doctor. I went once and he told me that I need an x-ray, but it costs £E 60. Where can I get that much money? He (her husband) sends the money to his mother and I can only save from the money my father sends me. If he (her husband) was here he would take me but my mother-in-law just says that I am sickly and that is my nature."

I asked Nagat why she went to the healer, an expedition which costs both time and money. She said that she was trying things within her means, and that one never knows what causes what. The healer had in fact prescribed some tablets, which we got from the pharmacy, for her infection. Women however do sometimes seek the professional help of a local healer to help them resolve the *mushahra*. These are people who possess the *mashahir*. The word *mashahir* implies the beings who cause the spell. It also implies the tools used by professionals to resolve it. These tools vary but always include a seashell, a necklace with various colored semi-precious, or not-so-precious stones, and a pharaonic-style human figurine. These figurines are described as *masakhit* (those who have been struck down by the wrath of God). They are believed to be representations of the ancient Egyptians who were struck down by God because they were nonbelievers. Indeed one of the most potent of *mushahra* breaking objects is the grave, corpse, or skeleton of a nonbeliever.

One healer with whom I very often visited used an old metal ashtray that had a pharaonic figure as a stand. The beads, shell, and figurines are stepped upon, passed around the body (down the neckline, over the chest, and out from underneath one's clothes) and were dipped in water, which is then drunk by the afflicted.

Mushahra explains much of the oft-noted confinement of new brides and mothers. It also establishes days for weddings and when it is safe for a mother to wean. Those planning to abort keep *mushahra* in mind. For example Farhana is a woman in her early forties. Her 17-year-old son died by electrocution when he was working in a building site in Helwan, outside Cairo. He was holding a cable when someone accidentally switched the power on. She was heartbroken by her loss. She was also pregnant. As a sign of grief she decided to abort the baby. As this was under discussion while we were paying our condolences, her cousin noted that it was the beginning of the month. "What am I, a young girl? What do I care if I never give birth again? Is there anything more to lose than the one that I have already lost?" exclaimed Farhana. A couple of days later she buried her fetus in a cavity in the wall of the house, as is the practice. Some months later she offered the aborted fetus to a woman who was seeking pregnancy. Crossing over aborted fetuses is another cure for the spell. Out in the desert there is another object of great potency. It is an ancient structure, which is now piled over with sand and resembles a small hill. It is built by the *masakhit* and believed to have their powers. Rolling down the side of it is thought to be a sure cure.

Mushahra is a familiar concept all over rural Egypt among both Copts and Muslims. It is unknown to well-to-do Cairenes, very few of whom have been able to abandon henna for brides and grooms despite a highly cosmopolitan self-image. The use of henna is similar to candles on birthday cakes and decorations on Christmas trees: vague in meaning but no one would dream of forgoing the ritual. In Cairo, new mothers are strongly advised to wear their diamond jewelry to deflect *mushahra*. Among educated Palestinian, Jordanian, Sudanese, and Moroccan women, the word *mushahra* strikes a distant and familiar bell.

While the above are personal observations, the literature on women and fertility in the Middle East concurs with these impressions. Under the heading 'Fertility Rites,' Blackman describes how peasant women in Asyut cure their infertility and how far apart they space their offspring (Blackmen 1927: 97–108). Many of the rites Blackman describes are still practiced today in the villages of Asyut. It is surprising to read the descriptions that Blackman gives of practices that involve the use of pharaonic amulets of cats, figurines, skulls, and deeply buried bones, in addition to other ritualized acts to counter bareness including lying on the railway tracks. To a large extent and with infinite variations, these rites are still practiced. However, *mushahra* beliefs provide a meaning-endowing framework within which these prophylactic and curative practices can take place. This framework is missing from Blackman's work, but so too is it missing from other ethnographies about Egypt and elsewhere, where the visible practices are described but not accounted for or explained.

In 1892, Abd al-Rahman Ismail included *mushahra* beliefs in his catalog of folk medical traditions called *Tibb al-rikka* ('The Medicine of Old Women') (Inhorn 1994). He describes *mushahra* as a collection of gems/stones strung together along with human forms of silver and gold. These human forms are known as *masakhit*, the term by which struck-down infidels are known. The woman who owns this object has the power to cure barrenness and eye disease (Ismail 1892: 13–6). In another section of the book he describes barrenness (*mushahra*) by eggplants. Under barrenness he also mentions the crossing over of a dead body as a famous old practice (42).

Partial record of *mushahra* can be found in the work of some anthropologists working in Egypt (most notably those of Ammar 1954; Abu-Lughod 1993a, 1993b; Harrison et al. 1993, Morsy 1980, 1982). The belief and practice is also known in the Sudan. In these texts the writers refer to the practices that infertile women resort to, and to the taboos that women who are fearful for their well-being must uphold. One finds passing references to the inauspiciousness of visitors coming from the graveyard and to the potent effects of railway tracks and red meat. On an even less specific level, one finds references to bridal and post-partum confinement in any text on the daily life of women in the region.

Mark Kennedy, who has written about *mushahra* among the Nubians in the south of Egypt is one of the first scholars to attempt to make theoretical sense of the spell and to transcend simple description. In an article titled "*Mushahra*: A Nubian Concept of Supernatural Danger and the Theory of Taboo," (1978) he puzzles at the diverse observances that come under the practice of *mushahra*. He interprets the spell in terms of the prophylaxis from malevolent water and death spirits who threaten fertility during periods of sacred vulnerability. He stresses the observance of taboos to please or neutralize spirits as the meaning-endowing framework by which *mushahra* is to be interpreted and intellectually represented (Kennedy 1978: 134; Inhorn 1994: 117).

Following similar reasoning, Janice Boddy presents a more elaborate interpretation of *mushahra* among rural north Sudanese women that also hinges on the concept of spirit possession. Boddy mentions *mushahra* as a kind of genital bleeding that is brought about by *mushahra*-afflicting substances and persons. She mentions gold jewelry as one such agent of the spell, describing how one woman, who was in labor but had no gold jewelry on, began to hemorrhage when her daughter entered the same room wearing a gold ring. She was cured when she was given the ring to wear. Placing these gold objects in water and looking at them can also cure an afflicted woman. This gold must be either Egyptian *bunduqi* gold (24–28 carat gold) or a Maria-Theresa coin (Boddy 1989: 313–4).

Boddy explains *mushahra* as a situation of violation of bodily integrity "caused by visually mixing experiential domains and in turn, by spirits attracted to female genital blood" (Boddy 1989: 106). Following the arguments of Mary Douglas on boundaries and the polluting potential of ambivalence, Boddy sees *mushahra* as a process of violation and reconstitution of significant boundaries (Boddy 1989; Inhorn 1994).

In her book on infertile women in Alexandria, Marcia Inhorn devotes a chapter to *mushahra*, which is known by the name of *kabsa* in Lower Egypt and in the coastal regions. She provides an elaborate, comprehensive, and detailed account of what she calls the *kabsa* complex. This is as yet the only work that has considered the spell and its practice with such depth and theoretical sophistication.

Inhorn's most significant contribution is that she shifts the focus from spirits to people. She posits the meaning of *kabsa/mushahra* in the polluting violation of boundaries. Reiterating part of Boddy's argument, she makes the connection between rooms and wombs (Boddy 1989: 105; Inhorn 1994). Both posit that when a woman's entrances are opened, i.e., by the flow of circumcision blood, defloration, or childbirth, the substitute boundaries that are reconstituted for the protection of her inner well-being, that is her fertility, are physical ones—they are the walls that surround her. If these physical boundaries are transgressed while her own natural guards are temporarily inoperative, then the transgressor's pollution reaches her. The only barrier between a woman who is vulnerable and the danger of infertility are the physical, ritually reconstituted, and socially maintained barriers around her.

Only polluting transgression can thus violate a woman. Inhorn lists pollution by blood, excreta, death, and wealth. The last is supposed to cover the effects that gold and jewelry are thought to have. In Alexandria she explains that women wear gold coins with the image of George V and other human forms on them, but this may be a representation of a different type of *masakhit* or infidel (Inhorn 1994: 127–8).

By stressing pollution over violation Inhorn points to the sharing of *kabsa* affliction and resolution among women. While women afflict one another, they also need one another's assistance in performing rituals of depolluting consubstantiality to affect a cure (132). She does mention rituals that preclude co-participants and which are performed with polluting substances or with a symbolic proxy. This is usually due to the inability of the afflicted women to find a willing co-participant. She then has to rely on an older officiant who advises her on how to perform the necessary rituals (144).

Inhorn's rich ritual analysis highlights the heterogeneous nature of the *mushahra/kabsa* complex. Women reproductively bound by the spell must overcome their binding by resorting to numerous venues and cures that may involve peers or professionals.

Further Interpretations

To the best of my knowledge, there is little else written about mushahra other than the works reviewed above. In the following section I would like to attempt further interpretations to compliment and engage the theoretical formulations written so far. There is no reason to contest the formulations that posit mushahra as a case of boundary violation. This is a coherent and reasonable argument, and one that is borne out by available ethnographic data. However this is a partial view of a very socially significant phenomenon. I would like to focus on the sociality of mushahra and its implications to individual and group identity by taking a closer look at liminal periods and liminality to address the function of mushahra beliefs in structuring the daily life of the community in which I worked.

The word *mushahra* derives its meaning form the Arabic word for month. In effect it refers to the actual and symbolic punctuation of time with the birth of the new moon. Each lunar month witnesses the roaming of the *mashaher*, which are the month-related spirits and spells. With the end of the month, the *mashaher* disappear and are replaced by those of the new month.

The moon plays a key role in the spell. A woman's liminality ends with the birth of the new moon. Indeed the moon plays a significant role in the lives of villagers on the whole. The single piece of information I did not have and which made me feel most like a hopeless outsider was knowledge of the moon. How I envied those who could look up into the sky and say, "Ramadan is in three days time." My excuse was that I lived in Cairo where the bright lights almost eclipse the moon itself. One woman teased me by saying, "You don't look up in Cairo *(Masr)*, do you?"

The Islamic calendar is a lunar one and it is incumbent on most villagers to be familiar with it. However, familiarity with the moon is more than a matter of knowing a calendar. It is an important dimension of social, and particularly female, life. Monthly cycles are reckoned by the moon. These are cycles that concern women. They keep track of their menstruation, due dates for delivery, and the early development of their children using this weekly and monthly calculation. Annual cycles are male affairs. The agricultural cycle, animal husbandry, and the weather are reckoned according to the Coptic calendar. In general, women are more familiar with the moon than men. It is common to hear a man ask his wife, mother, or sister when the beginning of the new month is.

The end of one month and the beginning of another is an instrumental time for matters other than reproductive binding. This is not a good time to wander outside the village. On questioning this injunction I was told that first of all it was dark! But aside from the practicalities, this interlude between months can effect mortal life in other ways. For some women it affects their cooking. During wheat harvests the annual supply of *kishk* is made. *Kishk* are balls of dried cracked wheat mixed with salted, sour milk and used as a cooking ingredient, snack, or as a condiment on long journeys. The production process takes at least a couple of weeks. Women hurry to finish before the end of the month because the next phase of the moon blackens and sours the *kishk*.

There are several theories that connect women and the moon. Buckley makes the most direct link by citing biological evidence to the effect that the full moon can emit enough photic stimulation for hormone release so that the new moon, which is born twelve to fourteen days later, is synchronous to the onset of menstruation in the case of some women (Boddy 1989: 101). I cannot claim that women in Upper Egypt are thus attuned to the moon. But I do think that *mushahra* belief conveys a view of the lunar cycle as being a complete one, and that the birth of the new moon signifies a clean start that is akin to the start of the monthly reproductive cycle of women.

According to Victor Turner, the moon is itself a liminal symbol. The waxing and waning moon is in constant transition; it is neither one thing nor the other but at the same time it is both (Turner 1974: 18). At another level, the moon is a familiar and reliable way for the timing of a woman's period of liminal vulnerability, which is at the same time a grace period when recuperating women rest.

I realize that I have offered indications of the instrumentality of the moon but no explanation. Frankly, I do not know what the symbolic, ritual, structural, or functional explanation could be. I have noted how the moon is observed. "Will you wean this month or the next?"; "Why have the wedding so early on in the month?"; and "Have you broken your palm reed charm or not, the moon is long gone?" are all questions I have repeatedly heard and noted. All I can comment is that since each women's liminality is an individual experience, marking time by the moon offers an assurance of some days of repose and a reliable means of keeping track of the time that lapses meanwhile.

Another overlooked aspect of the spell is its sociality. *Mushahra* absolves a woman, at least for some time, from the responsibility of her slow or unrealized pregnancy. But more important than the function of the spell as a temporary excuse is the leveling effect it has on women. Besides the relevance of people over spirits to the spell as noted by Inhorn, there is another very important social consequence to *mushahra*; it creates a constant channel of mobility from statuses of fertile to infertile and vice versa.

Evelyn Early, who wrote briefly on the topic in the context of other folk practices in urban Cairo notes that *mushahra* "(is a) socially induced situation . . . (that) . . . deflects the notion of a slow pregnancy from ego to another" (Early 1993: 105). This is a spell that can be cast on any woman by another. It places all women under the same rules, the same codes of practice. There is no differentiation. There is no initial state of well-being that predisposes one woman rather than another to having children. There is no essentially fertile or infertile woman.

Women are enjoined in a vulnerable liminality in which they partake at different times in their lives. At any given time, there are several women in a village or neighborhood who are *mushahra* prone or who can affect *mushahra*. As Early points out, "Almost everyday of her life, a married women is preoccupied with conceiving or avoiding conception, inducing or avoiding miscarriage, retaining health during pregnancy and lactation, undergoing safe delivery, nursing, or protecting her infant's health." This is the reality of the life of the majority of women. *Mushahra* provides one way of regulating the relationships between these women.

The concept of communitas may help to explain. Turner explains that communitas characterizes relationships between those jointly undergoing ritual transition. These bonds, he adds, are anti-structural in that they are direct, undifferentiated, and are outside structural relationships. In a more poetic vein he calls communitas "the sentiment of humanity" (Turner 1874: 274). Those who partake in *mushahra* belief and practice are in constant flux. They are in and out of periods of vulnerability and liminality in which they themselves are liminal beings. They represent the peculiar unity of the liminal in that they are both dangerous and in danger. But the relationships among them are characterized by common and empathetic understanding for it can happen to anyone at any time.

Turner describes liminality as "the Nay to all positive Structural assertions, (that is) in some sense the source of them all, and, more than that, is a realm of pure possibility whence novel configurations of ideas and relations may arise" (Turner 1987: 7). The individualized liminal positions of women suffering from or fearing *mushahra* is more than a period of structural suspension where normative values attached to being fertile or infertile are rendered inoperative. I would like to argue that it is the realm where probability is structured.

Women are not simply betwixt and between infertility for a limited period of time. The resort to *mushahra* as cure and prevention creates an arena where probability and potential are maintained in the face of simple assertions and bias. Women keep on trying to have children and go on pursuing cures and therapies in diverse medical traditions. Women travel distances in their pursuit of fertility, pool resources, and request the assistance of others. This may be, I propose, because *mushahra* provides a near endless sea of probability and with it the security of deflecting stigma from ego and serving to remind that all are vulnerable and that infertility, or slow conception are not far off hand.

There are many stories of mothers advising their sons to marry another wife. But the counter attack comes from anecdotes about such mothers who then lived to see their own daughters afflicted by *mushahra*. The moral of these stories is to remind audiences that "no one takes more than their given share."

That the woman bears the consequences of her inability to bear sons for her husband and his patriliny is an example of gender inequality. It is interesting to note however that in the context of Upper Egypt, and perhaps elsewhere, this inequality between men and women is mediated through same sex relationships, which are expressed as inequality among women. A man takes another wife, a mother shuns her daughter-in-law, and many other woman-to-woman gestures of hurt and harm. Where infertility is the instrument of a woman's oppression, *mushahra* provides an interesting commentary. True that many second wives bear the coveted son but there is an underlying theme to theses often tragic situations: it could happen to anyone.

Mushahra is one belief that enables women to take control of an uncontrollable and precious part of their lives; that is, their fertility and in some cases the health of their children (Early 1993: 108). Besides its symbolic and ritual interpretations, *mushahra* has a structural significance. It extends probability and potential to an arena of individual, family, and community life, which would otherwise be fraught with intolerable tension. One thing that demands attention is the degree to which *mushahra* may be 'unobserved but practiced.'

At one defloration ceremony I attended, I noted that the groom did not go back into the room with the bloodied kerchief. I felt a bit pleased since this was consistent with the practice in other such ceremonies and seemed to be directly related to *mushahra* aversion. But then hordes of guests started to flock into the bride's chamber as she sat still in considerable discomfort. All in all there were over sixty people singing and dancing in a very small room. Surely there must be someone there who could be a carrier of *mushahra*. Why were her female kin not concerned? Later on I was told: "Surely no one would be so mean as to enter her bridal chamber to harm her." But there were children, toddlers, dogs, and many women there! Perhaps it is more important to know that if the bride does not conceive, there are events to reflect upon and ways to diagnose the problem, but at such a lovely wedding and such a happy occasion no one was playing gatekeeper.

Conclusion

There are three major omissions in my paper. I have not considered the dominant theories of procreation in which upper Egyptians partake. I have also not considered male infertility, and I have overlooked the role of Islam. I shall briefly try to explain the relevance of *mushahra* to each of these issues.

Women do have a generative role in procreation. Despite the elegant argument put forward by Carol Delaney concerning Turkish villagers, it is difficult to agree with the notion of seed and soil she presents. It is true that "A woman is a vessel that empties," as one Upper Egyptian saying goes, and the language of reproduction in both English and Arabic, as well as in Turkish, is replete with the imagery of seed, fertile and barren land, and implantation or impregnation. However, "A boy takes after his maternal uncle" is another very common saying since the mother is a conduit for the genes of her own family. But verbalism aside, the visible practice of people counters this hegemonic language and analysis.

Insofar as male infertility is concerned, there is a necessary distinction that is made between male impotence and infertility. Folk and biomedical therapies are aggressively employed for the former. Indeed, one can interpret traditional defloration ceremonies as one way of saving men the embarrassment of a public display of possible impotence because the man uses his hands to deflower the bride and therefore does not have to prove his virility. Infertility however is recognized but is rarely seen as anything but temporary. Men may be slow in conceiving but rarely are they permanently incapacitated. The blame is put on the woman except if the man is clearly impotent.

As for Islam, it is unfortunate that Inhorn reaches out for another "dominant theoretical metonym," that of Islam, to explicate the significance of *kabsa/mushahra*. She links the Islamic concerns about cleanliness or bodily integrity and the perceived polluting effects of bodily emissions and fluids, which stress menstrual and postpartum blood, to the potency of polluting violations in binding the reproductive capabilities of women. *Mushahra* practices firmly place women outside the Islamic purity through which one gains access to God, notably through prayer and fasting, mainly because that which contaminates is also that which cures.

Mushahra is neither within nor outside Islam. It neither imitates nor opposes it. Ultimately practitioners of *mushahra* say, "God creates reasons *(rabbina biysabbib)*." God created the *mashahir* and created the danger of affliction. Thus women relieve themselves of any intimations of disbelief for all are strong believers. But when it comes to the use of clearly polluting substances, which women may wear internally or externally, or otherwise share, it is something else. It is neither a threat nor a challenge to religion or tradition. It is a practice that is un-Islamic if anyone takes the time to define it as such. It is this judgment of right and wrong that ensues from the use of the thick lens of Islam.

I hope to have avoided watertight explanations and pointed to an environment where the experienced insecurity of marginalized peasants is reflected in an ability to absorb and cope with uncertainty and maybe even to master an intellectual tool that helps those who need it.

In writing about *mushahra*, I was faced with a significant political problem. Can I write about such exotic, un-Islamic practices? What use is it? What does it explain? Who does it serve? I began to realize that this urge for self-censorship was not motivated by political correctness but rather by an attempt at ethnographic integrity. True that *mushahra* beliefs are sociologically significant and prevalent but I could not ignore the texture and sense of the whole issue. When going to borrow a skull from a neighbor or force-weaning puppies for later use, women were not engaged in a ritualized and solemn process. There was gossip, jokes, doubts, and even a fight anargument, when the neighbor refused us the skull.

Thus relaying the lived aspects of the spell seemed to be the only way of making it palatable. The commonsense aspect of *mushahra* lies in its value as an analytical tool, for it is thus employed by the women who practice it. It is a tool for expressing uncertainty and probability and one that espouses a basic justice (if I may be permitted an expansive word). As important as its rituals and symbols is its existence in the consciousness and world-view of women and of men. In the context of anthropological writing *mushahra* may be considered a paradigm which explicates ethnographic observations. In the context of the village, *mushahra* is a mental model that provides for possibility and for an expression of a kind of justice.

I started by wondering about women's toleration of pressures to prove their successful fertility. *Mushahra* is part, and a small part at that, of the strategies and practices women and men employ. In using the language of liminality I tried to focus not just on the practice of mushahra but on it bearing to relationships within the village. In discussing the contexts in which it operates, I tried to relay a sense of the grain of salt with which most strictures and norms are taken in an Egyptian village.

"*Mushahra* is all lies (*al-mashaher kizb*)," one woman told me. Meanwhile, we walked through a field of eggplants before crossing the three nearly unmarked graves of murdered corpses on a Friday afternoon, so as to resolve my own perceived affliction.

Bibliography

Abu-Lughod, Lila,1989, "Zones of Theory in the Anthropology of the Arab World," *Annual Review of Anthropology*, 18: 276–306.

———, 1993a, "Islam and the Gendered Discourse of Death," *International Journal for Middle East Studies*, 25 (2): 187–205.

———, 1993b, *Writing Women's Worlds: Bedouin Stories*. Berkeley: University of California Press.

Ammar, Hamed, 1954, *Growing Up in an Egyptian Village*. London: Routledge.

Ayrout, Henry Habib,1963, *The Egyptian Peasant*. Boston: Beacon Press.

Beck, L. and N. Keddie, eds., 1978, *Women in the Muslim World*. Cambridge: Harvard University Press.

Blackman, Winifred, 1927, *The Fellaheen of Upper Egypt*. London: George G. Harrap.

Bloch, Maurice,1992, "Birth and the Beginning of Social Life among the Zafimaniry of Madagascar," *Coming into Existence: Birth and Metaphors of Birth*, G. Aijmer, ed. 70–91. Gothenburg: IASSA.

———, 1991, "Language, Anthropology, and Cognitive Science," *Man*, 26: 183–198.

Boddy, Janice, 1989, *Wombs and Alien Spirits: Women, Men, and the Zar Cult in Northern Sudan*. Madison: University of Wisconsin Press.

Central Agency for Public Mobilization and Statistics (CAPMAS), 1993, *Egypt Maternal and Child Health Survey 1991*. Cairo: Center for Public Mobilization and Statistics.

Delaney, Carol, 1991, *The Seed and the Soil: Gender and Cosmology in Turkish Village Society*. Berkeley: University of California Press.

Early, Evelyn A., 1993, "Fertility and Fate: Medical Practices among Baladi Women in Cairo," *Everyday Life in the Muslim Middle East*, D.L. Bowen and Evelyn A. Early, eds, 102–108. Bloomington: Indiana University Press.

———, 1982, "The Logic of Well Being: Therapeutic Narratives in Cairo, Egypt," *The Ethnography of Health Care Decisions*. 16 (16): 1491–7.

Fernea, Elizabeth, ed., 1995, *Children in the Muslim Middle East*. Austin: University of Texas Press.

Harrison, Gail, et al., 1993, "Breast Feeding and Weaning in a Poor Urban Neighborhood in Cairo, Egypt: Maternal Beliefs and Perceptions," *Social Science and Medicine*, 36 (8): 1063–69.

Hinds, M. and El-Said Badawi, 1986, *Dictionary of Egyptian Arabic*. Beirut: Librairie du Liban.

Inhorn, Marcia, 1994, *Quest for Conception: Gender, Infertility, and Egyptian Medical Traditions*. Philadelphia: University of Pennsylvania Press.

Ismail, Abd al-Rahman, 1882, *Tibb al-rikka (The Medicine of Distaff)*. Cairo: al-Matba'a al-Amiriya.

Kennedy, John,1978, "'Mushahra': A Nubian Concept of Supernatural Danger and the Theory of Taboo," *Nubian Ceremonial Life*, John Kennedy, ed., 125–145. Berkeley: University of California Press.

Mascie-Taylor, G.N., 1993, *The Anthropology of Disease*. Oxford: Oxford University Press.

Mernissi, Fatma, 1985, *Beyond the Veil: Male-Female Dynamics in Modern Muslim Society*. London: Saqi Books.

Morsy, Soheir, 1978, "Sex Roles, Power, and Illness in an Egyptian Village," *American Ethnologist*, 5 (1): 137–151.

———, 1980, "Body Concepts and Health Care: Illustrations from an Egyptian Village," *Human Organization*, 39 (1): 92–96.

———, 1981, "Towards a Political Economy of Health: A Critical Note on the Medical Anthropology of the Middle East," *Social Science and Medicine*, 15B (2): 159–163.

———, 1990, "Political Economy in Medical Anthropology," *A Handbook of Theory and Method in Medical Anthropology*, J. Johnson and C. Sargent, eds., 26–46. Westport: Greenwood Press.

———, 1993, *Gender, Sickness, and Healing in Rural Egypt: Ethnography in Historical Context*. Boulder: Westview Press.

Rassam, Amal, 1980, "Women and Domestic Power in Morocco," *International Journal of Middle East Studies*, 12: 171–179.

Rosen, Lawrence, 1989, *The Anthropology of Justice: Law as Culture in Islamic Society*. Cambridge: Cambridge University Press.

Tucker, Judith E., ed., 1993, *Arab Women: Old Boundaries, New Frontiers*. Indianapolis: Indiana University Press.

Turner, B., 1991, "Recent Developments in the Theory of the Body," *The Body, Social Process, and Culture Theory*, M. Featherstone, M. Hepworth, and B. Turner, eds., 1–37. London: Sage Publications.

Turner, Victor, 1967, The Forest of Symbols. Ithaca: Cornell University Press.

———, 1968, *The Drums of Affliction: A Study of Religious Process Among the Ndembu of Zambia*. Oxford: Clarendon Press.

Conclusion
The Medical Cultures of Egypt

HANIA SHOLKAMY

The Importance of Being Healthy

Management of a sickness event implies the mobilization of all accessible intellectual, social, and material resources. The individuals and
families discussed in this book's chapters look to the past for reasons
and cures, mobilize relationships to acquire access to therapy and
support, and expend in cash and in kind to survive the event and min-
imize their losses. The essays in this volume describe the dynamism
of health management and protection in Egypt. Each entry describes
how networks are forged, resources are pooled, and effort is spent to
tide over the disease conditions or meet health and fertility aspirations.
Such processes, when initiated to confront 'serious' conditions, are
always collective and inscribed in memory as a moment of
significance.

By way of conclusion, this essay considers the medical cultures of
Egypt as reflected in the theoretical contributions of researchers.
Despite the existing wealth of ethnographies and articles there is still
room for a volume such as this, not only to confirm health and ill-health
as dimensions of social life, but to further our understanding of this
changing society. This short essay presents a critical analysis of the
space in which further work is needed and argues for the continued
importance of research in medicine, society, and culture.

The medical cultures of Egypt have fallen victim to the fluctuating
interests of academics and researchers. The surge of interest in the
1980s and early 1990s has petered down to a trickle of concern about

bioethics, Islam, and a narrow range of medical procedures such as in vitro fertilization, elective and selective embryo termination, organ transplants, and the definition of medical death.[1] The most notable recent addition to the medical anthropology of Egypt is Marcia Inhorn's work on assisted fertilization (Inhorn 2003).

But what does existing work tell us about the social life of Egyptians? Anthropologists have selected a narrow set of theoretical idioms to answer this question. But lurking in the studies of local or native health/medical cultures, which tend to orientalize and perhaps inadvertently devalue the beliefs they describe (Ismail 1892; Blackman 1927; Kluzinger 1878; Kuhnke 1990), and in the valuable ethnographies of health as social practice (Morsy 1993; Nelson 1971; Inhorn 1994) and the reports, articles, and policy papers aimed at policy makers, donors, and those working in the field of health and development are assumptions and insights on Egyptians and the society they are so dynamically creating.

The social world of embodied conditions can help inform and interrogate assumptions about diseases but also perceptions of Egyptian society. Describing social processes through the lens of embodied experiences and conditions is an undervalued tool of social analysis. It is unfortunate that the field of health has worked itself into an interdisciplinary ghetto that is becoming policy- and program-oriented. While this may conceivably lead to informed policy, it is simultaneously depriving social research of a wealth of ethnographic knowledge. It is indeed surprising how little is known of the medical cultures of Egypt. It is even more lamentable to realize how outdated and stereotypically 'traditional' existing knowledge tends to be. The relevance and tenacity of non-western, non-biomedical, and seemingly non-rational therapies and practices remain unsituated in modern social life. The authors are contributing such a situation and maintaining the focus on health as a priority for people. The essays also make clear the essentially social dimensions of health, disease, and health-seeking behavior, which make manifest the importance of social knowledge to medical care.

---

1. Publications in this field are slowly materializing. Sherine Hamdy is an Egyptian anthropologist working on donor transplants. The University of Bochum in Germany is sponsoring a research project on bioethics, Islam, and medical technologies.

A cursory reading of 'traditional medical beliefs' makes clear the domination of a limited number of culturally distinct root paradigms in the analysis of ethnographic observations. Medical anthropologists have chosen the idioms of Islam, humeral medicine, or spirit possession to analyze medical practices and beliefs.

Islam

Islam has been used as a broad meaning-endowing framework with reference to which a variety of therapeutic and prophylactic practices have been 'intellectually' justified to the reading audience. While practices such as the belief in jinn and the efficacy of written charms are sanctioned by Islam, they are not a product of this faith. Inhorn chooses to cite the rules of Islamic pollution and absolution to explain fertility and infertility beliefs. But the uses of Islamic knowledge about health take place at a much more conscious level. They are expressed in the tradition of forbearance and fortitude with a much wider prevalence than has been noted by anthropologists who chose the lens of Islam for their studies. Ali notes the discourse of Islamic sanctions and prohibitions concerning family planning. But who resorts to the scriptures when considering their reproductive intent, and why and when they do it are questions left unanswered in much of the literature (Ali 2002).

Prophetic medicine, particularly cupping (hadjam), is witnessing a strong revival here in Egypt. This method combines cupping and cauterization/scarring to draw and let 'bad blood.' The Prophet himself is acknowledged to have practiced this form of therapy, which relies on its own anatomical construction of the body (Encyclopedia of Islam). There is an official religious decree (fatwa) from Dar al-Iftaa (no. 764/1995) issued in response to a request asking whether or not the use of Qur'anic verses and hadjam are sanctioned. The fatwa makes reference to three prophetic traditions to argue that the Prophet resorted to hadjam:

Vol. 7, Book 71, No. 603:
Narrated Jabir bin 'Abdullah: I heard the Prophet saying, "If there is any good in your medicines, then it is in a gulp of honey, a cupping operation, or branding (cauterization), but I do not like to be branded (cauterized)." (author's translation)

Vol. 7, Book 71, No. 602:
Narrated Ibn 'Abbas: The Prophet was cupped on his head for an ailment he was suffering from while he was in a state of ihram (ritual cleanliness in preparation for pilgrimage) at a water place called Lahl Jamal. Ibn 'Abbas further said: Allah's Apostle was cupped on his head for unilateral headache while he was in a state of ihram. (author's translation)

Vol. 7, Book 71, No 595:
Narrated Ibn 'Abbas: The Prophet was cupped and he paid the fees to the one who cupped him and then took medicine that is sniffed (su'ut). (author's translation)

Cupping has currency in modern Egypt. A generation of providers follow aseptic procedures, rely on a map of the body that specifies the pressure points for various ailments, and ask patients to sign an informed consent form before treatment (something physicians often forget to do!).[2]

Hadjam is an important part of the medical traditions of ancient Arabia. Along with some basic surgical procedures, herbal antidotes, and medications, the use of cauterization and incense was practiced long before the time of the Prophet. This old Arabic medicine relied in large part on the principles of humeral medicine or on the belief in spirits and omens. However, cupping in particular was favored and used by the Prophet and has not only outlived other therapies, but is periodically given new interest and revived thanks to this prophetic association.

There is an important distinction to be made between *hadjam* as a therapy that refers to the Prophet's traditions and other therapies to which researchers have added the adjunct of Islam. The difference lies in the devotional aspect of these therapies. Cupping and similarly sanctioned therapies prescribed by the Prophet Mohammed are practiced as a medical therapy and religious act, which inscribe faith and submission on the body of the believer. Other therapies or beliefs such as the resort to *jinn* or to written charms are not devotional. Researchers may locate exegesis that notes the celestial structures of Muslim scriptures and the primacy and sanctity of the written word but that is perhaps not the

---

2. Unfortunately documents explaining modern *hadjam* are unpublished. A source of information is a pamphlet written by an anonymous, self-taught practitioner: *al-Hadjama ikyas al-hawa' al-haditha: kayf tatjannab naql al-'idwa.*

choice or the conscious explanation of those resorting to these therapies. Soheir Morsy's description of Islamic clinics negates the Islamic nature of the science but illustrates the use of Islam to sanction the quality of the service. These clinics are usually organized as part of the outreach services of large mosques. This service is perceived to be of high quality and is often free or heavily subsidized. This is the link between the medical service and Islam. But the therapies, medications, and science on which both rest is purely biomedical, often aggressive, and proud to be undifferentiated from biomedical services in secular institutions (Morsy 1988). These clinics provide welfare services with a measure of success that state health services have failed to do. They are arenas where clients contest the hegemony of the state. Frequenting Islamic clinics is not a devotional act but a political one.

There are clearly three elaborations on Islam as a paradigm for understanding health-related behavior. One relies on Islamic traditions and heritage and is devotional, another relies on the ethics and political organization of Muslims, and a third can be explained by reference to the cultural components of Islamic societies and scripture.

A frequent reference that Egyptians themselves make to Islam when experiencing hardship and disease is about acceptance and resignation. Muslims will not challenge the will of the Almighty to inflict ill-health and hardship. This gesture of faith may create passive patients and rife territory for medical malpractice and health mismanagement. Indeed, Egyptians have by and large put up with a measure of both.[3] However the function of faith in extending social and psychological relief and succor should not be neglected or unappreciated.

The late 1990s have confirmed the solid facts concerning the social determinants of disease (Wilkinson and Marmot, 1998). Out of the ten acknowledged determinants,[4] three focus on social cohesion, social inclusion, and social support. In Egypt, religion plays a major role in all three aspects of social life. We could perhaps add faith as a social determinant of health and health-seeking behavior, and so break the hold of research that views Islam as a political force, a resource of traditional practices, or a set of structures and rules.

---

3. This statement reflects the opinion and experiences of the author. It is also based on interviews with members of the medical syndicate committee on malpractice, who preferred not to be named.
4. They are hierarchy, stress, care in early life, social exclusion, work, unemployment, social support, addiction, diet, and transportation/environment.

Using the notion of social determination does not assume that the linkages necessarily produce good health. On the contrary, it is proposed as a critical endeavor that could operationalize the potential of health studies to dig deeper and get closer to peoples' social lives.

Humeral Medicine

The medical ethnography of Egypt has also been analyzed practice in terms of these principles of humeral medicine.[5] The language of humors is spoken by most villagers in Upper Egypt. Cauterization is said to be effective in the cure of a variety of conditions. A person with a temper is described as having 'hot blood,' and someone who is heartless or humorless is said to have 'cold blood.' Lay medical diagnosis often refers to 'cold in the stomach' and 'heat in the head.' However these utterances and practices in themselves are not indicative of a humeral medical system.

Evelyn Early has tried to analyze Cairene women's therapeutic choices in humeral terms, transcending food and substance classification to examine the value of balance. She calls the health system she is examining the

---

5. Humeral medicine as elaborated by Hippocrates, Galen, and Ibn Sinna (Avicenna) is now a two-millennia-old medical paradigm characterized by simplicity and uniformity (Foster 1994: 2). It is a tradition that locates health in balance and equilibrium, and which explains ill-health in terms of disequilibrium suggested by naturalistic not personalistic causes. It has been incorporated in what has become known in Egypt as *al-Tibb al-Nabawi*, which is also distinguished by its naturalistic etiology. It also relies on a significant knowledge of the nature of the afflicted individual, that is, the natural complexion of the patient (sanguine, phlegmatic, bilious, melancholic) as these complexions imply states of body and mind. Moreover seasonality and activity are crucial to diagnosis and therapy (Foster 1994: 7, 43). There is an assumption that humeral medical beliefs survive in Egypt. Soheir Sukkary-Stolba, for example, in writing about food classifications and child diet, chose to interpret the emic distinctions of light and heavy food as ones which correspond to categories of hot and cold as constructed by humeral food classifications (Sukkary-Stolba 1987). But as Soheir Morsy notes, for rural Egypt, people's food classifications tend to correspond to actual properties of food relating to its thermal not metaphoric heat and digestibility (Morsy 1993: 297).

baladi system.[6] She locates the principles of this *baladi* physiology in the ideal of the natural functioning of the body. Any irregularity, either in physiological sequence or in social relationships, assumes etiological significance. Balance is defined not in terms of humors but in terms of a conception of what is normal *(tabi'i)* and concordant with the pragmatism of everyday life (Early 1988: 73–81).

But balance can also be a purely pragmatic construct. Mothers who have given birth must eat from everything because they are weak and have lost much blood. Shock *(khar'a)* knocks the breath of life out of its victims, so they need cautery to shock them into recovery. Too much sugar for children can make them sick. All these calculations rely on a direct cause-and-effect rationale and not a symbolic one of humors and their interactions. However, yearning and jealousy can also damage health. Jealousy and fright, according to this concept of health determinants, are as real as chemicals and protein deficiency. All upset the body and leave it prone to disease.[7]

Balance, both natural and social, is key to the medical system of Egypt. Indeed health cannot truly exist in the midst of excesses. Hania Sholkamy writes of infertility spells acting as breaks on the euphoria of fertile women. Montasser Kamal questions the possibility of perceived good health in the midst of economic disparities. Employment opportunities and authorities also act as health determinants in the same way. In the new language of the World Health Organization, this tension between health and hierarchy is called "The Social Gradient."

Most diseases and causes of death are more common lower down the social hierarchy. The social gradient in health reflects material disadvantages and the effects of insecurity, anxiety, and lack of integration (Wilkinson and Marmot, 1998: 8).

The modern discourse on public health reminds the wealthy that overeating and lack of exercise are unhealthy; it reminds policymakers that the underprivileged and poor are placed in a structural position of ill-health. The principle of balance, as socialized in Egyptian medical cultures, echoes this modern wisdom.

---

6. The term *baladi* derives from the word *balad*, which means 'country' in Arabic. *Baladi* means 'my country' and denotes the urban, unwesternized poor.
7. A notion legitimized by biomedicine once it discovered the function of the hypothalamus.

The World of Spirits

The third paradigm that figures in the analyses of health and healing in Egypt, as elsewhere, is spirit possession. The zar cult is a familiar form of exorcism that persists in Egypt today. It is expressive of a firm belief in the parallel and sometimes pernicious world of spirits. Spirit possession and exorcism have intrigued medical anthropology and provided a root paradigm for analyzing cosmology and health beliefs. In some studies, possession itself has been explicated in terms of gender relations of domination and patriarchy (Morsy 1988), as a means of escaping confinement and domination (Early 1988), and as an idiom of somatization that is of cultural essence to the Middle East (Nelson 1971). Exorcism has also been compared to 'folk psychotherapy' (Boddy 1989: 353). In a rich symbolic analysis of the zar cult in north Sudan, Janice Boddy argues that it is a means by which women counter their cultural over-objectification. Exorcism ceremonies become a means by which women "step outside the world and gain perspective on their lives" (354).

But spirit possession is invariably isolated from other roles played by spirits in the lives of men, women, and children. For example, in Egypt, the prevalent belief in the powerful role of the sister spirit (*qarina*) is not separate from the belief in domination by other spirits. The sister spirit is most active during the first forty days of an infant's life and is the potential cause for infant or neonatal mortality. But children are rarely possessed when older. This does not mean that the spirits exorcised by *zar* and those that afflict children are unrelated or have no bearings on one another.

The most significant aspect of this medical culture is not its acknowledgment of a parallel spirit universe. This is a medical system that overwhelms the world of spirits through its concern for the relationships between human beings in this world. This is made clear by the contribution of Heba El-Kholy to this volume. These relationships define health and ill-health and even use spirits to affect and structure these definitions. Envy (*hasad*), sister spirits, and *mushahra* are all supernatural expressions of social relationships. These various strands of analytical thinking leave many questions unanswered. Why are spirit-possession beliefs and sister spirits beliefs unarticulated? Why does the literature mention an Egyptian equivalent of sickness by fright (*susto* in Spanish) without attempting to understand the emic physiology or anatomy on which it is based? Why don't children get possessed? Why can men resist their own sister spirits? *Zar* is irrelevant to children because they are not immersed in the kind of sexual relationships often related to spirit possession. Children don't get possessed because they are not in a social position that permits such possession. Disparate snatches of medical practice can become varied dimensions of a medical culture if this essential generative role of social relationships is acknowledged.

There are another two approaches to health management in Egypt. Both are socially informed and situated. Morsy has masterfully described the politics of powerlessness as expressed in bodily conditions (Morsy 1993). This volume rests on the foundations built by her work to describe how people not only express their predicaments but also their social selves and perceptions of the world (Morsy 1993: 5; see also Young 1982). Her politico-economic approach situates disease in the nexus of poverty and powerlessness, which increase the risks and liabilities of sufferers. Hind Khattab, on the other hand, adopts the languages of modernization theory by describing access and utilization to reproductive health services, also in terms of power relations but ones that need knowledge and education to create a balance and beneficence (Khattab 2000). Both approaches describe the relationship between poverty, powerlessness, gender, and disease. Morsy locates panacea in empowerment. Khattab's remedy is confined to health messages, physician training, and improving quality of care.

The essays in this volume are at the threshold of a complementary but slightly different approach. They describe health and the body as sites of active agency and not as the playground of other forces such as tradition, belief, ideology, and socioeconomic need. The essays posit the individual as a conscious agent forging self and identity as well as social positions and knowledge through the process of health management and the pursuit of bodily ideals and aspirations. These acts can gesture personal change, social mobility, and newfound beliefs, or the assertion of existing ones. They do so in active ways and their effects may be temporary but they are still significant for our understanding of society and culture.

The medical cultures of Egypt are more than the product of the confluence of hardship and poverty. Neither are they structured by symbolic gestures alone. They present a cacophony of practices that have a contextualized coherence. Each episode of resort is an active choice that changes the person making the choice.

The Logic of Protection and Prophylaxis

Key to understanding the multiplicity of medical cultures is the study of prophylaxis and protection. Indeed no understanding of Egyptian medical cultures is possible without reflection on the logic of protection. Envy and envious agents are at the heart of this logic of protection. Diseases, accidents, loss of appetite, wasting and stunting, and other mishaps are recognized as dangers but are perceived to be manifestations of a much more serious danger, that is, the envy and ill wishes of others. The look or gaze (*nazra*) and person (*nifs*) lead to sickness, weakness, or misfortune. "He got diarrhea from underneath a gaze" is a common explanation given by parents. The diarrhea is the visible condition but what really caused it? Why that child and not his sibling or neighbor is a question whose answer necessitates a higher order of causation (Sholkamy 1995). This order of causation reflects that interconnectedness of the individual and the set of relations in which he or she exists. *Nazra* and *nifs* cannot exist outside of community. Bad intentions can only come from another human being who is in a position to comment and thus envy another. Parity is a prerequisite to envy (Ghosh 1982: 222). One can only be envied by another who perceives themselves to be equal in some respect and therefore entitled to the same good fortune as the person envied (Blackman 1927; el-Aswad 1988; Kluzinger 1878; Ghosh 1982: 222).

But the eye is only a symbol and a medium. The underlying conceptualization of human relations in which the eye is instrumental is based on the principle of equality. The logic of envy is that people are or believe they should be equal to each other. A person's lot in life should be like everyone else in the community. Consequently when blessed, a person must either hide the blessing or emphasize a problem so as to counteract the imbalance caused by a blessing. Here again a clear expression of social and functional balance as a virtue is made. A true belief in the expectation of equality provides understanding for unwilling and unintended envy. These practices shield from those who are at a disadvantage and therefore cannot help but seek, even if impetuously, to redress the imbalance. "The eye does not choose" as the saying goes, but the imperative of equality drives it to cause harm.

The intellectual distance between biomedical prophylaxis and connected protective practices suggest that we are discussing separate worlds with separate concerns. This distance would seem to advance the stereotypical dichotomy between local beliefs as irrational ideas that are contingent on supernatural considerations and biomedical principles that are rational and scientific. But the difference between the two approaches to prevention can also be interpreted in terms of their concern for different levels of causation. Biomedicine's focus on immediate dangers to health contrasts with theories that attempt to explain the process by which these immediate dangers select certain individuals and not others.

The issue of the selective behavior of many diseases is one which biomedicine has neither solved nor succeeded in dismissing. Indeed, it is one that is imposing itself on the biomedical research agenda. Currently it is accepted that many diseases are affected by genetic predisposition. Genetics are also pointing to the individualized nature of disease and affliction. In a sense, research on the 'cocktail' of genes that predisposes one person to obesity, another to hypertension, and a third to specific kinds of cancer is also saying that while environmental factors matter, they impact some individuals more than others. It implies that diseases are selective because genes catalyze the interaction and culminate in different results according to the genetic constitution of each person.

There is a similar argument at the heart of beliefs concerning personal disposition defining one's exposure to ill-health. Here, as in modern theories of genetics, personal circumstances or personal constitution interact with environment to render one healthy or unhealthy. The vitality of personhood and circumstance create a vernacular rendering of the biomedically-constructed rationality of genetics. The remote similarity lies in the fact that these two sets of traditions and beliefs attempt to answer some of the same questions.

Non-biomedical models of health and disease seem to have far preceded medical ones in the recognition of the social determination of ill-health. Now that public health researchers have come up with evidence to prove this wisdom, recognition is due as to how locals constructed and protected health in terms of social values and experiences. Researchers are not trying to measure, calibrate, and understand how such social experiences and perceptions structure health and the predisposition to ill-health.

Hasad is neither distinctively rural nor Egyptian. It is not exclusively Islamic, since beliefs in 'envidia' exists in many communities in South America. The importance of mentioning envy in the context of a discussion is its indication of the relationship between health, ill-health, and the principles which organize social and political life.

The old and wise say that ultimately all things, both good and bad, come from God *(Rabbina biysabbib)*. However this belief does not translate into apathy, fatalism, and a feeling of powerlessness as far as believers are concerned. That God is the ultimate source of all incidents, initiatives, and events is a belief that helps those who have suffered or lost loved ones to accept the tragic or difficult trial. However, until the 'deed has been done' believers are enjoined to strive to protect themselves and seek remedies and redress. God, as the ultimate source, is a formula that helps *ex post facto* acceptance but is not one which precipitates an *a priori* fatalism. It is a tenet that leaves plenty of room for people to take initiative in defining, managing, and protecting their health and well-being.

It is surprising that medical anthropologists have not taken on the challenges of local protection despite the importance of preventive medicine. Although charms, amulets, incense, blue stones, and other tools of protection have been described and documented exhaustively, the intellectual and social implications of this logic are less considered. The essays in this volume have considered protection and the positive pursuit of health ideals in the context of modern Egypt. It is through these reflections that identity and the individual's place in the world is constructed and enacted. Prevention, recognized as a mainstay of modern medicine, is also the foundation of the individual's social and cultural interactions with diseases. The essays in this collection echo this concern to establish its relevance to self and health and not to question or argue the efficacy or rationality of nonbiomedical prophylaxis.

Future Linkages between Medicine, Society, and Research

> They have their ideas. Many children come in with a *higab* (protective amulet) on their chests. This is very common. Or a small child comes in wearing black so that he or she lives. Even the underwear is black. The *galabeya* is black and they wrap him in one of their veils so that the baby lives. They do other things for treatment. They say they stung or cauterized him. I've seen cauterization on the back. I do not know what it is for. . . . One here hears many of these things. When you know this you appreciate that it is difficult to communicate! (Egyptian physician from Cairo working in Asyut as quoted by Sholkamy 1997: 257)

The social character of health and sickness warrants more attention from audiences beyond the attentions of medical anthropology. Of urgency are the promotion of medicine as a social science and the immersion of health services in social and cultural contexts.

Anthropologists have established the link between culture, medicine, and health well but have not communicated this wisdom to healthcare providers, consumers, or decision makers. Lip service to this cause has become common but its realization and impact remain rare.

The case for better communication between provider and patient is expressed in the quote above. Communication requires understanding and that can only take effect if there is mutual respect. The Reproductive Health Working Group (RHWG) in Cairo is an inter-disciplinary network of researchers and clinicians who are attempting to promote this understanding. It is under the nurturing care of this group that this volume was born. Group members have been writing across disciplinary lines and carrying out research along multidisciplinary ones to realize this objective.[8]

This collection is part of a wider effort to make the medical and the social mutually significant and relevant. There are two fronts on which we wage this campaign. One arena is social research, where health topics seem to be theoretically and intellectually limited to those who are involved in the pragmatics of healthcare. The second is the medical sphere in which medicine is still constructed as a universal and historical science and practice.

The fragmentation of social life into interlocking spheres such as family, economy, politics, and religion has been a function of the ever-growing specialization of social sciences. Old ethnographies used to take on all spheres at once. Newer ethnographies which detail practices and perceptions with all the nuances of what is said and unsaid, done and not done, are obliged to focus on one arena of life to make the task of description manageable. To understand the dynamics of health and describe its structure requires truly multidisciplinary approaches. It also describes an expansion of scope that encompasses and integrates personal, social, political, medical, and economic domains. Such old-style but medically informed ethnographies are in short supply.

But health and its pursuit is occupying more and more of people's lives and resources. In the absence of effective insurance systems, the prospect of ill-health or disability looms large as a major risk to the survival and viability of families and individuals. The quality of public

---

8. The Reproductive Health Working Group has a long list of monographs and a policy series that addresses both healthcare providers and researchers, and which is published in both Arabic and English.

health services is still compromised by a number of factors including poor regulation and constant efforts to keep costs low. The focus on reproductive health and family planning affects the ability of health services and providers to give care for other maladies and needs. The statistics available support this analysis. Of the total expenditure on healthcare in Egypt, 53.9 percent is private, implying that more than half of patient needs are not covered by public services. Of that amount only 0.5 percent comes from prepaid plans and the other 49.6 percent is out of pocket (WHO 2001). So while health and the risk of disease are becoming more central to social life, they are receding from the horizons of social studies.

A relatively recent health measurement has been devised by the World Health Organization (WHO) to measure life expectancy with an adjustment for time spent in poor health. This indicator measures the equivalent number of years a newborn is expected to live, in full rather than compromised health. Healthy life expectancy (HALE) is a proxy for the estimation of people's propensity to become seriously ill by nationality. Although it has been an often-criticized measurement, it is useful in enabling researchers and health planners to reflect on the likelihood of ill-health occurring in a population.

The figures claim that men in Egypt lose 13.7 percent of their life expectancy and women lose 16 percent as a result of ill-health. These figures are not high per se, or as compared to the rest of the world. These measurements imply that while on the whole men and women are living longer, they are not doing so in good health. World populations are either suffering from the diseases of poverty, which are mostly communicable diseases precipitated by deficient resources, poverty, lack of sanitation, primary healthcare, and clean water or from the non-communicable diseases of wealth associated with over-eating and inactivity, such as cardiovascular diseases, diabetes, and cancers. Egypt has a mixed population suffering from both kinds of morbidities.

Despite the constant drive of biomedicine to standardize health globally and develop measurements that define optimal health, there remain cultural and historical variations on how people experience health and ill-health. Health researchers have discussed somatization as the way in which we express or embody instances of disruption or stress. People somatize in different ways. But the influence of culture and society goes beyond the provision of our language of distress. Our toleration of disease conditions, expectations of ourselves, and aspirations towards health and well-being are socioeconomically and culturally constructed.

Mothers in developed countries may be well aware of the dangers of antibiotic overuse and happy to manage childhood fevers in the good old-fashioned way, but in developing countries mothers may view cold compresses and fluids as the predicament of the poor who cannot afford a course of potent pills (Sholkamy 1995).

In this volume Farha Ghannam describes the cultural flows that influence women's pursuit of beauty and ideal body weight. Women's expectations and aspirations are shaped by place, class, education, resources, family, and taste. Perhaps recognized morbidities afford less cultural and personal latitude yet the work of Hind Khattab (2000) shows how toleration of disease burdens and recognized symptoms is likewise socially defined. The multiplicity of resources and beliefs that people access in order to mange health also confirms the relevance of the social to the medical, and the medical to the social.

The main therapeutic options are public and private medical clinics and hospitals, ethnomedical specialists, and community members who have one form of expertise or another. These three resources instruct and contradict one other intellectually and materially in a number of ways. All are employed by their ultimate consumers seeking to make the most of available resources. Health is structured and defined in terms of one medical culture locally defined, one which retains a heightened sense of social and political context, but is restored and managed through recourse to a variety of medical services and traditions. In use of biomedical services the men and women mentioned in this volume see the tradition of western biomedicine as one that has the clout of modern science, the magic and mystery of drugs and medications, and the prestige of the urban middle class. They use biomedicine because it provides a shortcut to relief from distressing symptoms but they may not necessarily rely on the cognitive structures upon which medicine relies to define health and ill-health. While this eclectic use of health and medical resources has often been cited and commented on, less has been said about the implications of these medical idioms to the structuring of identity and linking individuals to society, and society to the world. The essays presented here see medical idioms as forces that forge social ties and identity.

But the meanings of practices and beliefs associated with health have not been theoretically exhausted. Indeed they have not been considered at great depth and the changes in such behavior have gone unnoticed. Tradition is blamed for many mishandled disease conditions. Egypt, as historians tell us, has had a long history of 'modern' biomedical services, including public health campaigns and initiatives (Fahmy 1998; Kuhnke 1992). Egypt was modernized by Muhammad 'Ali in the nineteenth century, then by the British occupation in the mid-twentieth century, then again by Abd al-Nasser. With each wave of modernization, medicine, public health, and medical services featured as important components of ideological and political campaigns. Not enough effort has been invested in excavating and deciphering such a rich body of perceptions and beliefs. Medical practitioners and policy makers retain the middle-class bias of describing locally constructed medical etiologies and locally available resources for addressing them as 'superstition,' which can be dispelled by the strong medicine of modern science. Such an unsatisfactory dismissal does not help to explain why these beliefs persist.

It is important to historicize and study the practice of medicine. It would be a worthwhile effort to make manifest the social and cultural assumptions of health service providers and decision makers. It would be fascinating to know what providers think they know about their work and their clients. The essays at hand do not assume such an undertaking but they do make clear the potency and power of social perceptions to health and to the embodiment of diseases and disabilities.

The thee of this volume is that observers of Egypt cannot only know more about heath by considering culture, but become more in tune with culture by looking at how people manage their health. There is scope and promise in linking health, self, personhood, sociality, and material resources in a manner that engages readers, health professionals, and observers of a vibrant and changing Egypt.

Bibliography

Ali, Kamran Asdar, 2002, "Introduction," *Planning the Family in Egypt: New Bodies, New Selves*. Cairo: The American University of Press.

El-Aswad, S. 1988, *Patterns of Thought: An Anthropological Study of Rural Egyptian World Views*, Ph.D. dissertation, University of Michigan.

Banerji, D., "The Place of Indigenous and Western Systems of Medicine in the Health Services of India," *Social Science and Medicine*, 15A: 109–114.

Blackman, Winifred, 1927, *The Fellaheen of Upper Egypt*. London: Georg G. Harrap.

Boddy, Janice, 1989, *Wombs and Alien Spirits: Women, Me, and the Zar Cult in Northern Sudan*. Madison: University of Wisconsin Press.

Collier, J. and S. Yanagisako, eds., 1987, *Gender and Kinship*. Stanford: Stanford University Press.

Early, E., 1988, "The Baladi Curative System in Egypt," *Culture, Medicine and Psychiatry*, 12: 339–348.

Fahmy, K., 1998, "Women, Medicine, and Power," *Remaking Women*, L. Abu-Lughod, ed., 35–72. Princeton: Princeton University Press.

Foster, George McClelland, 1994, *Hippocrates' Latin American Legacy: Humoral Medicine in the New World (Theory and Practice in Medical Anthropology and International Health, Vol 1)*. London: Routledge.

Ghosh, Amitav, 1983, "Relations of Envy in an Egyptian Village," *Ethnology*, 22(3): 211–223.

Gibbs, H.A.R., B. Lewis, Ch. Pellat, C. Bosworth, et al., eds., 1960–2002, *The Encyclopaedia of Islam*, 2nd edition, 11 vols. Leiden: E.J. Brill.

Inhorn, M., 2003, *Local Babies, Global Science: Gender, Religion, and In Vitro Fertilization in Egypt*. New York: Routledge.

———, 1996, *Infertility and Patriarchy: The Cultural Politics of Gender and Family Life in Egypt*. Philadelphia: University of Pennsylvania Press.

———, 1994, *Quest for Conception: Gender, Infertility, and Egyptian Medical Traditions*. Philadelphia: University of Pennsylvania Press.

Ismail, Abd al-Rahman, 1892, *Tibb al-rikka (the Medicine of Distaff)*. Cairo: al-Matba'a al-Amiriya.

El-Katsha, Samiha, S. Watts, 2002, *Gender, Behavior, and Health: Schistosomiasis Transmission and Control in Rural Egypt*. Cairo: The American University in Cairo Press.

Khattab, H., N. Younis, and H. Zurayk, 1999, *Women, Reproduction, and Health in Rural Egypt: The Giza Study*. Cairo: The American University in Cairo Press.

Kluzinger, Karl B., 1878, *Upper Egypt: Its People and its Products*, 1st ed. New York: Scribner, Armstrong & Sons.

Kuhnke, Laverne, 1990, *Lives at Risk: Public Health in Nineteenth Century Egypt*. Berkeley: University of California Press.

Lane, Sandra, Jok Madut Jok, and Mawaheb T. El-Mouelhy, 1988, "Buying Safety: The Economics of Reproductive Risk and Abortion in Egypt," *Social Science and Medicine*, 47(8): 1089–1099.

Morsy, Soheir, 1980, "Health and Illness as Symbols of Social Differentiation in an Egyptian Village" *Anthropological Quarterly*, 53 (3): 153–161.

———, 1988, "Islamic Clinics in Egypt: The Cultural Elaboration of

Biomedical Hegemony," *Medical Anthropology Quarterly*, 2 (4): 355–369.

———, 1993, *Gender, Sickness, and Healing in Rural Egypt: Ethnography in Historical Context*. Boulder: Westview Press.

Nelson, Cynthia, 1971,"Self Spirit Possession and World View: An Illustration from Egypt," *International Journal of Social Psychology*.

Sholkamy, Hania, 1995, GOBI-FF, "Strange Names and Amulets: The Logic of Protection in Rural Upper Egypt," Arab Regional Population Conference, Cairo, December.

Sukkary-Stolba, Soheir, 1987, "Food Classifications and the Diets of Young Children in Rural Egypt," *Social Science and Medicine*, 25 (4): 401–405

As-Sunnah Foundation of America, http://www.sunnah.org, accessed 2003.

Tabishat, M., 2000, "Al-daght: Pressures of Modern Life," *Situating Globalization: Views from Egypt*, Cynthia Nelson and Shahnaz Rouse, eds., 203–230. Bielefeld: Transcript/Verlag.

WHO, 2001, World Health Organization health statistics: http://www.who.org, accessed 2003.

Young, Allen, 1982, "The Anthropologies of Illness and Sickness," *Annual Review of Anthropology*, 11: 257–285.

Wilkinson, R. and M. Marmot, 1998, *Social Determinants of Health: The Solid Facts*. Geneva: World Health Organization.

About the Authors

Heba El-Kholy is a development practitioner and social anthropologist with a Ph.D. from the University of London's School of Oriental and African Studies (SOAS). For the past twenty years, she has been working in the field of social development in Egypt and the Arab world with a range of national, bilateral, and international organizations, focusing on gender issues, poverty alleviation, and micro-enterprise development. She is currently senior regional officer at the United Nations Development Program (UNDP) in New York.

Farha Ghannam is an assistant professor of anthropology at Pennsylania's Swarthmore College and is a member of the Reproductive Health Working Group. She is the author of *Remaking the Modern: Space, Relocation, and the Politics of Identity in a Global Cairo* (University of California Press, 2002).

Montasser M. Kamal is a medical doctor and anthropologist with extensive experience in the field of public health and medical anthropology. He is one of the founding members of the Arab Forum for Social Science and Medicine. Currently working in Canada, he is a member of the Reproductive Health Working Group.

Hania Sholkamy is an assistant professor with the Social Research Center and the Forced Migration and Refugee Studies Program at the American University in Cairo. She was program associate at the Population Council and is a member of the Reproductive Health Working Group.